Your H
in Youi
Horosce

C000244061

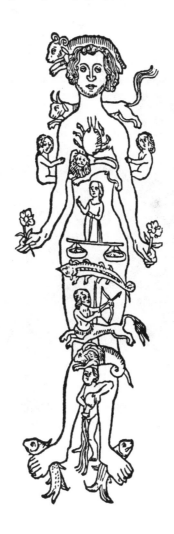

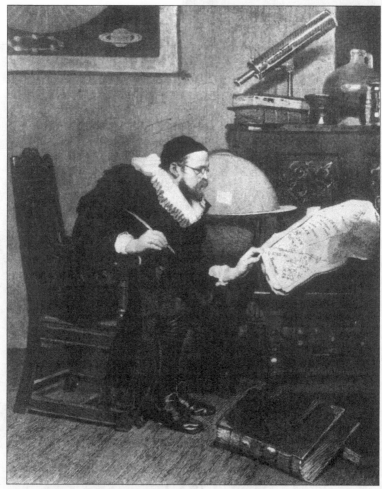

The Astrologer. Engraving from the late 19th century by Joseph Deman-
nez, after John Seymour Lucas.

Your Health
in Your
Horoscope

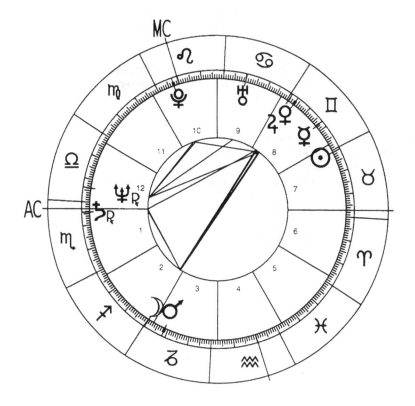

Introduction to Medical Astrology

Stefan Stenudd

arriba.se

Stefan Stenudd is a Swedish author, artist, and historian of ideas. He has published a number of books in Swedish as well as English, both fiction and non-fiction. Among the latter are books about astrology, the cosmology of the Greek philosophers, the Japanese martial arts, and an encyclopedia of life force concepts.

His novels explore existential subjects from stoneage drama to science fiction, but lately stay more and more focused on the present. He has written some plays for the stage and the screen. In the history of ideas he studies the thought patterns of creation myths, as well as Aristotle's *Poetics*. He is also an aikido instructor, 6 dan Aikikai, Vice Chairman of the International Aikido Federation, member of the Swedish Aikikai Grading Committee, and the Swedish Budo Federation Board. He has his own extensive website:

www.stenudd.com

Also by Stefan Stenudd:
Life Energy Encyclopedia, 2009.
Qi: Increase Your Life Energy, 2008.
Cosmos of the Ancients: The Greek Philosophers on Myth and Cosmology, 2007.
Aikido Principles, 2008.
Attacks in Aikido, 2008.
Aikibatto: Sword Exercises for Aikido Students, 2007.
All's End, 2007.
Murder, 2006.

Stefan Stenudd's Astrology Website:
www.horoscoper.net

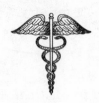

Your Health in Your Horoscope: Introduction to Medical Astrology.
Copyright © Stefan Stenudd, 2009
Book design by the author.
All rights reserved.
ISBN: 978-91-7894-021-9
Publisher: Arriba, Malmö, Sweden, info@arriba.se
www.arriba.se

Contents

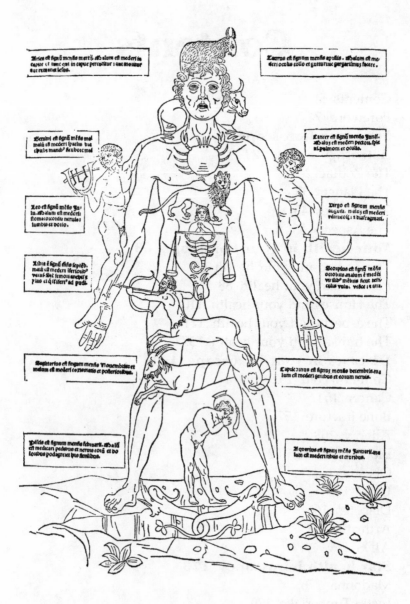

Zodiac Man, or Astrological Man, showing the relations between the Zodiac signs and the body parts they are traditionally said to govern. This is used in medical astrology. From Fasciculus Medicinae by Johannes Ketham, 1494.

Your Health in Your Horoscope

Foreword

Please, do not use this book instead of medical expertise to guard your health! That's not what it is intended for, and that's way beyond its reach.

I wrote this as an introduction to the age-old principles of medical astrology, the tradition of searching for clues about one's health in the horoscope and in the movements of the planets in our solar system. Had these systems been perfected, we would have cured a lot of diseases way before modern science found remedies for them. We did not.

Astrology is not a science, but a tradition that we could call metaphysical, another way of looking at the world and our lives than the methods developed by modern natural science. It cannot substitute science any more than science can incorporate astrology.

The best use you can have of this book, except as an introduction to this field of astrology if you have a general interest in it, is to serve as an alternative way to contemplate your health and its issues. This different perspective might help you to gain insights into the complexity of living your life in ways that agree with you the most.

If you like, you can try some of the suggestions given in the book, to see if they might improve your well-being – but do so only if your doctor approves of it, or if it's self-evident that it can in no way cause you any harm. Never let it interfere with the advice or treatments suggested by professional physicians.

I cannot stress this enough.

That said, I do person-
ally believe that astrology
can actually help you find
ways to improve your well-
being, either directly by
what your horoscope reveals
about your health issues, or
indirectly by making you
think in new ways about
your life and habits, and
thereby discovering circumstances that you had previ-
ously been unaware of or
underestimated.

Any method of contem-
plation, even one as odd and
mysterious as astrology, can
increase your self-awareness
and your understanding of
yourself. That's probably the
best use you can make of
your horoscope. See it as a
strange mirror for an alternative self-observation.

Apart from that, it's fascinating to get familiar with
thoughts and symbols that
have been around since the
dawn of civilization.

Stefan Stenudd

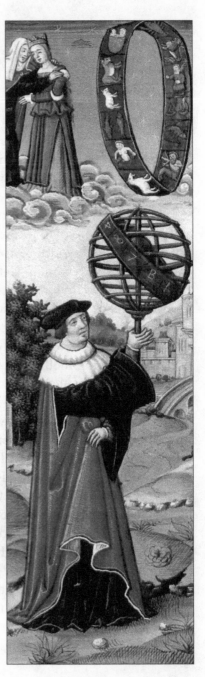

Your Health in Your Horoscope

Your own horoscope

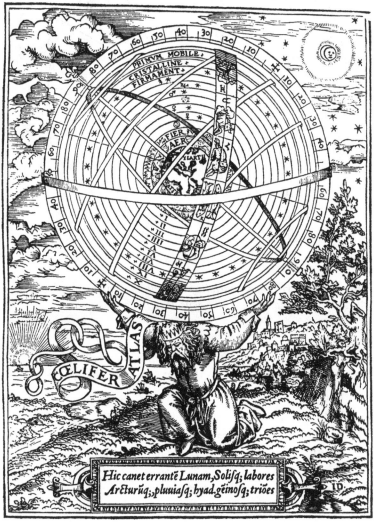

Atlas, carrying the whole world on his shoulders. Woodcut from The Cosmographical Glasse by William Cunningham, 1559.

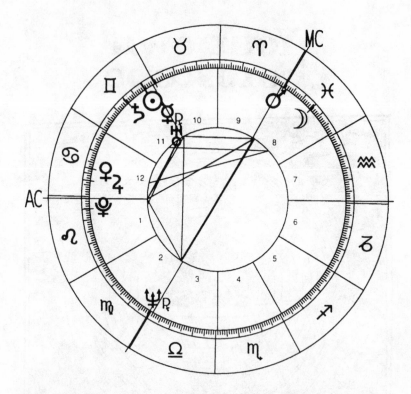

Horoscope. A birth chart (nativity) with all its components: the Zodiac, the Houses, the planets, and the aspects.

☉	Sun	♈	Aries, the Ram
☽	Moon	♉	Taurus, the Bull
☿	Mercury	♊	Gemini, the Twins
♀	Venus	♋	Cancer, the Crab
♂	Mars	♌	Leo, the Lion
♃	Jupiter	♍	Virgo, the Virgin
♄	Saturn	♎	Libra, the Scales
♅	Uranus	♏	Scorpio, the Scorpion
♆	Neptune	♐	Sagittarius, the Archer
♇	Pluto	♑	Capricorn, the Goat
AC	Ascendant (AC)	♒	Aquarius, the Water Bearer
MC	Medium Coeli (MC)	♓	Pisces, the Fishes

Your Health in Your Horoscope

Your own horoscope

The age old system of astrology has found a great assistant in the modern computer. With it, calculating a horoscope chart works like a charm. Before the computer there was a lot of work needed, and the astrologers used *ephemerides*, thick books with planet positions listed in tables. Now, you enter your birth data in a simple computer screen menu, and have the result in less than an instant. Anyone can do it.

If you're interested in charting more horoscopes than your own, you may want to purchase an astrology program to install on your computer. One of them, *Astrolog*, is free of charge, but the others usually cost more than $100, in some cases twice or three times that sum.

But if you just want to find out the details of your own birth chart, it can be done for free on a number of websites, such as *Astrolabe* and *AstroDienst*.

What you need to know

This is what you need to know, in order to get your precise birth chart:

1   Your birth date.
2   The time of your birth.
3   The place of your birth.

Birth date

Your birth date can be no problem. Day, month and year. The menu of the chart calculator website or computer program will be clear about how to enter that information.

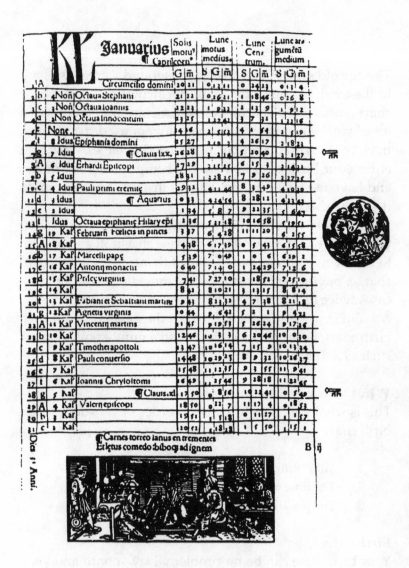

Calendar with the positions of the sun and the moon in the Zodiac, on
each day of a month, by Johannes Stöffler, 1518.

Your Health in Your Horoscope

Time of birth

The time of your birth should be as exact as possible – to the minute. That can be tricky. Some hospitals record the birth time as a routine, others not. Mothers should not be trusted to remember it with any accuracy. They were quite preoccupied at the time.

Be suspicious of a birth time on the hour, like 6 AM or 4 PM, also something like 6:30 AM or 4:15 PM. If you come across an odd time, like 6:28 AM or 4:14 PM you can probably trust it to the minute. A birth time given as 6:25 AM is probably something between 6:23 and 6:27, which is close enough.

For most things in the horoscope, a few minutes make almost no difference at all. Watch out with the Ascendant (AC), Medium Coeli (MC), and the House cusps, though. They have a mean movement through the Zodiac of 1° in 4 minutes – sometimes faster, sometimes slower. The moon has a mean movement of 13° a day, so it takes a lot of minutes for the moon to move significantly. The other components of the horoscope are much slower.

If you don't know your birth time at all, make a horoscope chart for 12:00 PM – midday. That way, the horoscope cannot be more than 12 hours wrong. Of course, that's far too much when it comes to the AC, the MC, and the House cusps – so you have to do without those in your chart, until you find out your birth time.

There are astrological methods for figuring out a birth time. You check *transits* and *progressions*, which are methods of prediction through planetary movements in relation to the birth chart, and compare those to significant events in your life. Thus, you sort of go the reverse way to establish your birth time.

I am not too fond of that method, since it demands a trust in astrology before it can prove itself. Also, there is

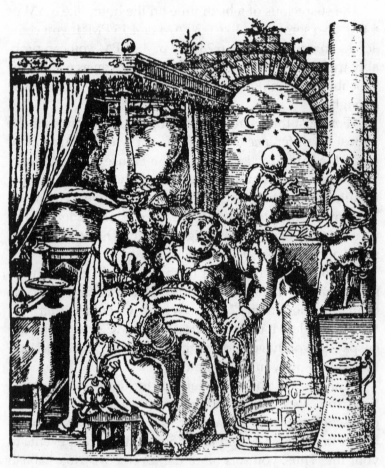

Astrologers by the window study the stars in the sky at a delivery. This kind of astrological attention was exclusive to royalties and the aristocracy. Woodcut from De Conceptu et Generatione Hominis by Jacob Rueff, printed in 1587.

Your Health in Your Horoscope

much room for misunderstanding, since transits and progressions sometimes work in mysterious ways.

You do better to use some detective work to find out your actual birth time.

Place of birth

The place of your birth is probably as well known to you as the date is. You don't need to be more precise than the city – or the nearest town, if you were born in the countryside. Don't bother to calculate the exact position of the hospital where you were delivered. Ten kilometers make almost no difference in the chart, nor do 20 or 30.

Observe that the longitude (east-west distance measured from Greenwich in England) makes slightly more difference than the latitude (north-south of the Equator). Still, don't worry about anything less than, say, 30 kilometers.

Most computer astrology programs have lists of thousands of cities, their longitude and latitude, so you rarely need to check that yourself.

There is one oddity with latitude. In the polar regions, beyond the arctic circles (latitude 66°23.5' North and South), the astronomical formulas can't really calculate the Ascendant. It is done with approximations and some other tricks. Astrological computer programs do it without hesitation – their manuals should reveal why and how. Anyway, if you're born in a polar region, you should consider this.

Chart types

The internet resources and computer programs have slightly differing designs, but their calculation results should be identical. Much bigger differences are to be found in the many kinds of horoscope charts there are to choose between – in any horoscope software. There are many options, some of them quite cryptical and confusing to anyone but the most knowledgeable astrologer. If you're not sure about what choices to make, do like with any computer program: stick to the default options.

Except for pure differences in design, these are the most significant alternatives for horoscope charts:

1   House system.
2   Planets and astrological points to include.
3   Aspects and their orbs.

House system

The House system is the way the twelve astrological Houses are calculated. The most common systems are *Placidus* and *Equal House*. In Placidus, a system made known in the Renaissance, the Houses have differing sizes, and the MC is the cusp of the 10th House. In Equal House each House is the same 30° in size, and MC can be in any House from the 7th to the 12th. Both systems (and any other system worth considering) have the AC as the cusp of the 1st House.

I have the impression that Placidus is the most commonly used House system. Me, I prefer Equal House for a number of reasons. It relates logically to the Zodiac, where each sign is also 30°, it adds nuance to the MC, it is mathematically more sound – and it's the oldest, used already by the Greek mathematician Ptolemy, who wrote *Tetrabiblos*, the classic book on astrology, in the 2nd century.

What you should do, though, is to compare the two systems on your horoscope, and decide for yourself which one fits you the best.

Planets and astrological points

Planets and astrological points to include are numerous, if you allow them all. These are the basic ones, on which all astrologers agree:

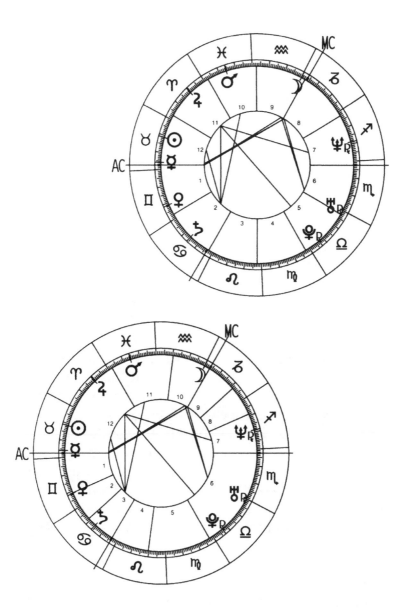

Horoscope of the English soccer player David Beckham in two versions: the top is with Equal Houses, the bottom with the Placidus House system. Notice the different sizes of the Houses in the latter. These differences can vary considerably, depending on the time and place of the birth.

Planets

☉	Sun
☽	Moon
☿	Mercury
♀	Venus
♂	Mars
♃	Jupiter
♄	Saturn
♅	Uranus
♆	Neptune
♇	Pluto
AC	Ascendant (AC)
MC	Medium Coeli (MC)

In addition to those, the lunar nodes – *Dragon's Head* and *Dragon's Tail* – are quite often used. Some use *Chiron*, a celestial body discovered in 1977, and some add asteroids, fixed stars, mathematically calculated points, and so on.

Which ones to use? In addition to the basic twelve on the list above, stick to the ones you are familiar with and have found valuable to include. Again, use your own horoscope as a guinea pig to reach your own conclusions.

I recommend that you start with only the twelve listed above. They are quite a handful to interpret, so you are in no hurry to complicate your horoscope additionally, before being well acquainted with them. Also, they are without a doubt the most important and influential ones.

Aspects and orbs

Aspects and their orbs have their default values in any horoscope computer program, but most of them allow for the user to adjust these values. There are five basic aspects, used already by Ptolemy:

Aspect		Angle
☌	Conjunction	0°
☍	Opposition	180°
△	Trine	120°
□	Square	90°
✳	Sextile	60°

A majority of astrologer would agree that those five aspects are the most important. In addition, some use the *quincunx*, 150°, which is by some regarded as quite powerful, and the weaker *semi-sextile*, 30°.

The orb is the number of degrees allowed for an angle to be marked as an aspect in the horoscope. For example, a 10° orb makes anything between 110° and 130° a trine. Of course, the bigger the orb, the more aspects in a horoscope. It is common for astrologers to use different orbs for different aspects – a big one to the strongest aspects, the conjunction and opposition, and a small one to the weakest, the sextile. In any case: an aspect is more important if it is close to exact.

I use rather small orbs – something like 4° for all aspects. I do so because you tend to look at relations between planets anyway, whether they are actually in aspect or not, so you need to have the close ones pointed out clearly. There's no need to make a cobweb of the chart.

Zodiac signs

The Zodiac signs, star signs, are the most well-known components of the horoscope. They are twelve:

Zodiac signs
♈ Aries, the Ram
♉ Taurus, the Bull
♊ Gemini, the Twins

♋ Cancer, the Crab
♌ Leo, the Lion
♍ Virgo, the Virgin
♎ Libra, the Scales
♏ Scorpio, the Scorpion
♐ Sagittarius, the Archer
♑ Capricorn, the Goat
♒ Aquarius, the Water Bearer
♓ Pisces, the Fishes

They are usually counted from Aries to Pisces, as above. Aries is the sign the sun enters at the Spring Equinox – in past times this was regarded as the beginning of the year. Your own star sign is simply the sign where the sun was at the time of your birth. Of course, the other planets and astrological points of the horoscope can be in any other Zodiac sign.

Western astrologers never alter the Zodiac signs. They are always the same as with Ptolemy, and even before his days. Other cultures, though, have different names for them, but most astrological systems have a similar division of the sky into twelve equal sectors.

Free horoscope charts online
Here are some websites with free horoscope calculations:

www.alabe.com
www.astro.com
www.0800-horoscope.com
www.astro-software.com
www.abacusastrology.co.uk

And here is a free astrology program for your computer:

www.astrolog.org

Astrology basics

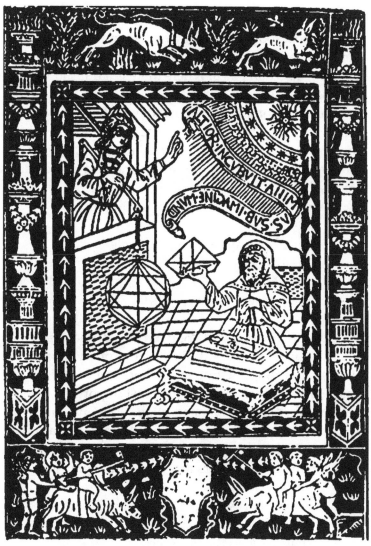

Astrologer calculating planetary positions with an astrolabe. Illustration from Annulus Astronomicus by Bonetus de Latis, c. 1493.

Astrology basics

The foremost tool of astrology is the horoscope, a chart of planetary and other celestial positions at a certain time, as seen from a certain place. Where there is a time and a place, a horoscope chart can be made.

The most common one nowadays is the birth chart, or nativity, based on the time and place of a person's birth. But horoscopes can be made for other things as well – countries, companies, projects, as long as a time and place can be established.

There are four components of a horoscope:

1   The planets and astrological points
2   The 12 Zodiac signs
3   The 12 Houses
4   The aspects

Western astrology is clear on the Zodiac signs and Houses, but astrologers differ on how many planets and aspects (angles) to include in the horoscope. Still, there is consensus on which ones are the most important.

Now, the four components above each give the answer to a particular question, regarding events and characteristics in the life of the person whose horoscope chart is studied. These are the four answers that the components give:

1   Planets and astrological points show *what* to expect.
2   Zodiac signs show *how* to expect it.
3   Houses show *where* to expect it.
4   Aspects show *why* to expect it.

More about this is explained in the chapters about these components. Observe that the only active forces in the horoscope are the planets and astrological points. The other components just describe, locate and explain these forces.

Geocentric

In the horoscope chart, the above components are marked at their respective positions, as seen at the time and place of the horoscope in question. The perspective is *geocentric*, i.e. as seen from Earth – although in reality the planetary movements are *heliocentric*, orbiting around the sun. What matters in astrology is how the sky looks from our viewpoint.

Charts

There are many ways to design a chart. In old Greece as well as the rest of Europe up until recent times, the most common way of drawing the horoscope chart was the so-called envelope design, where each triangle of the figure represented an astrological House. See the horoscope of Martin Luther on the next page.

Nowadays, the circular horoscope chart is used by all astrologers. In it, the outer circle marks the Zodiac, where each of the twelve Zodiac signs is 30° of the total 360° circle. They are placed in a counter-clock order. Inside of that circle, the positions of the planets are marked. Also, there is the twelve part division of the astrological Houses. The aspects between planets are marked with straight lines between them.

See the modern style circular horoscope chart on the next page.

The Ascendant (AC), the *Rising point* in the east, should be at the left side of the horoscope, and Medium Coeli (MC) somewhere on the top half of the horoscope. That means the horoscope's east is to the left, its west to the right, its south

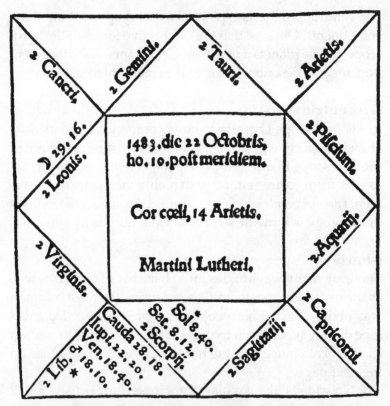

The horoscope chart of Martin Luther (1483-1546), made with the envelope design that was the standard in the Renaissance. Each triangle represents a House, with the cusp of the 1st House (the Ascendant) to the right, marked as 2° Virgo (Virginis). The planets are placed in the Houses they occupy, with notes on their degree in the Zodiac sign. The Equal House system is used.

is up and its north is down. The horizon is represented by a line from the Ascendant to the Descendant at the opposite side of the horoscope. So, what can actually be seen of the sky at the time and place of the horoscope is only what is above that line.

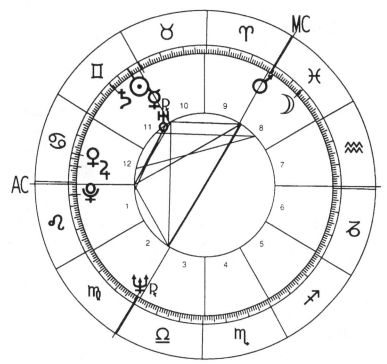

A circular horoscope chart, which is used by all modern astrologers, although with some differences in design. The place of birth is in the middle of the circle, and the horizon is the line of the Ascendant to the cusp of the 7th House. The lines in the innermost circle mark the aspects.

Reading

In astrology, the components above are interpreted in a combined way. A planet, its Zodiac sign, its House and aspects – they are all brought together in the search for the specific meaning in the horoscope. That is not an easy task, and astrologers may come to different conclusions – although they agree on most of the basics.

The Zodiac

In astrology as well as astronomy, the Zodiac is a 360° circle around the Earth, where each of the twelve Zodiac signs is 30°. In astronomy it is simply used as a coordinate system, to mark the positions of celestial bodies. In astrology, though, it is much more.

In the horoscope, each Zodiac sign represents a character, a tendency, which affects any celestial body therein. In that way, the Zodiac signs give the *how* to events and circumstances indicated by the horoscope.

Every planet moves through the Zodiac, and changes character according to what sign it is in. The planets are the acting forces in the horoscope, but the Zodiac signs nuance and alter their character.

Here are the twelve Zodiac signs, their English meanings, and keywords for their respective characters:

Zodiac signs		*Keywords*
♈	Aries, the Ram	challenging, impulsive
♉	Taurus, the Bull	conservative, concrete
♊	Gemini, the Twins	communicative, playful
♋	Cancer, the Crab	caring, sensitive
♌	Leo, the Lion	dominant, proud
♍	Virgo, the Virgin	careful, minute
♎	Libra, the Scales	negotiating, ethical
♏	Scorpio, the Scorpion	hidden, passionate
♐	Sagittarius, the Archer	impatient, independent
♑	Capricorn, the Goat	ambitious, decisive
♒	Aquarius, the Water Bearer	profound, original
♓	Pisces, the Fishes	searching, submissive

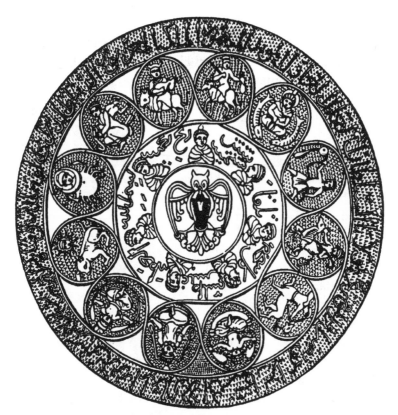

Arabian Zodiac from the 13th century.

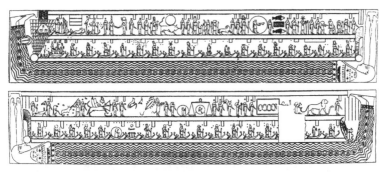

Egyptian Zodiac from the temple of the goddess Hathor in Dendera, 2nd century CE.

Motto

Each sign can also be said to have a *motto,* an expression that helps to clarify its character. Here are the mottos of the twelve Zodiac signs:

Sign	Motto
Aries	"I am."
Taurus	"I have."
Gemini	"I think."
Cancer	"I feel."
Leo	"I want."
Virgo	"I scrutinize."
Libra	"I balance."
Scorpio	"I wish."
Sagittarius	"I see."
Capricorn	"I use."
Aquarius	"I know."
Pisces	"I believe."

Element and quality

The characters of the Zodiac signs are to a large extent dependent on their *element* and *quality.* Every sign belongs to one of the four Greek elements, which represent four sides of life:

Element	Type
Fire	action
Earth	making
Air	thinking
Water	feeling

Since there are twelve signs and four elements, there are three signs belonging to each element. There are also three different basic qualities that signs have:

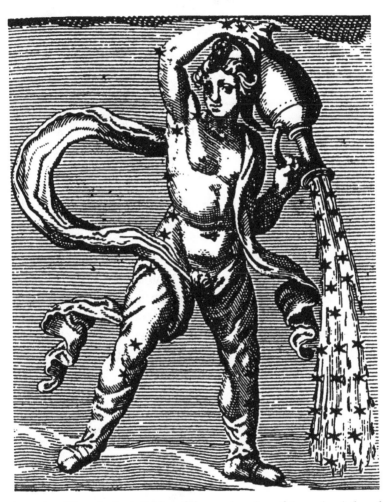

Aquarius. The astrological idea of the coming Age of Aquarius is based on the movement of the Spring Equinox backward through the Zodiac. It has moved through Pisces for the past 2000 years, and will enter Aquarius during the next couple of hundred years. There is little agreement among astrologers as to when, exactly. Some say that it has already happened.

Introduction to Medical Astrology   29

Quality	Type
Cardinal	leading
Fixed	static
Mutable	following

So, each sign has its own combination of element and quality:

	Fire	Earth	Air	Water
Cardinal	Aries	Capricorn	Libra	Cancer
Fixed	Leo	Taurus	Aquarius	Scorpio
Mutable	Sagittarius	Virgo	Gemini	Pisces

In principle, the combination of element and quality that is unique to each sign, decides what its character is.

Ruling and exalting

Each Zodiac sign is also said to have a *ruling* and an *exalting* planet. This simply means that some planets are particularly enforced by the character of that sign. A planet rules over the Zodiac sign where it fits better than the other planets do, and it exalts in a sign where it fits better than any other planet than the ruler of that sign.

Here are the ruling and exalting planets (note that also the sun and the moon are regarded as planets in this context, as is Pluto, in spite of its recent degradation):

Sign	Ruler	Exalted
Aries	Mars	Sun
Taurus	Venus	Moon
Gemini	Mercury	Jupiter
Cancer	Moon	Venus
Leo	Sun	Pluto
Virgo	Mercury	Venus

Libra	Venus	Mercury
Scorpio	Pluto	Neptune
Sagittarius	Jupiter	Uranus
Capricorn	Saturn	Mars
Aquarius	Uranus	Saturn
Pisces	Neptune	Mercury

Since there are twelve Zodiac signs and only ten planets to divide between them, Venus and Mercury both rule and exalt in two signs each.

Regarding what planets rule and exalt in what signs, astrologers don't agree completely, but most of the above is generally accepted. In any case, the rulership and exaltation should not be overly emphasized in horoscope interpretations. A planet's character in a sign speaks well for itself, without these generalizations.

Star sign – the sun

When people are said to be born in a certain Zodiac sign, it only means that the sun was in that sign at their birth. It's their sun sign. The sun is only one component in the horoscope – although an important one – so predictions based only on this are not astrologically adequate. The whole horoscope has to be considered.

The sun moves steadily through the Zodiac signs, spending about 30 days in each of them. The calendar system of leap years makes the dates of change from one sign to another jump around a little, but in average, these are the dates that the sun spends in each sign:

Sign	Sun transit
Aries	March 21 – April 19
Taurus	April 20 – May 20
Gemini	May 21 – June 20

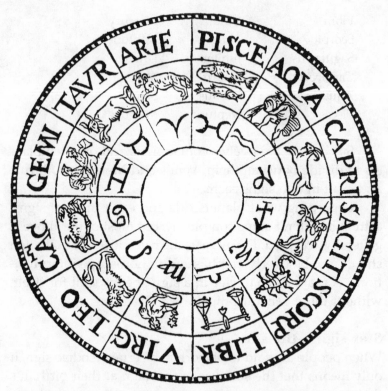

The Zodiac, its images and symbols. Illustration from Cosmographia by Franciscus Barocius, 1585.

Cancer	June 21 – July 22
Leo	July 23 – August 22
Virgo	August 23 – September 22
Libra	September 23 – October 22
Scorpio	October 23 – November 21
Sagittarius	November 22 – December 21
Capricorn	December 22 – January 19
Aquarius	January 20 – February 19
Pisces	February 20 – March 20

Your Health in Your Horoscope

If you are born on a date of change, or the day before or after it, you should have your sun position calculated by a horoscope program, to ascertain what sun sign you are.

Spring equinox

The traditional order of the Zodiac signs starts with Aries, because it is the moment of the spring equinox. That date was also the first day of the new year in ancient Europe. At the fall equinox, the sun moves into Libra. At the summer solstice it enters Cancer, and at the winter solstice Capricorn.

Symbols

The symbols used for the Zodiac signs are the same in astrology and astronomy. Here is a strict rendering of them:

♈ ♉ ♊ ♋ ♌ ♍ ♎ ♏ ♐ ♑ ♒ ♓

Zodiac symbols. From left to right: Aries, Taurus, Gemini, Cancer, Leo, Virgo, Libra, Scorpio, Sagittarius, Capricorn, Aquarius, Pisces.

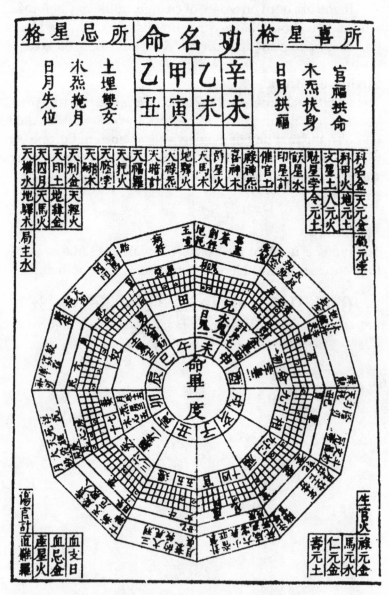

Chinese horoscope from the 14th century. There are many similarities between Chinese and Western astrology, but the former stresses the importance of Jupiter more.

Your Health in Your Horoscope

The Planets

In the horoscope, each planet represents an acting force, either internally in a person or externally in the world. The planets are the only active components in the horoscope. The Zodiac signs, the Houses and the aspects give character and setting to them, or link them together – but only planets generate action. In that way, the planets give the *what* to events and circumstances indicated by the horoscope.

Not all of those objects that are grouped as planets in the horoscope are actual planets in the astronomical meaning. The sun and moon are included, although one is a star and the other a satellite to Earth. Pluto is still regarded as a planet in the horoscope, and a powerful one at that. Also included are the Ascendant and Medium Coeli, although they are no celestial bodies at all.

The *Ascendant* (AC) is the rising point of the Zodiac on the eastern horizon, which is why it is also called *Rising* or *Rising Sign*. *Medium Coeli* (MC) is the highest point of the Zodiac, therefore also called *Midheaven*. They have their counterparts in the *Descendant* (DC) and the *Imum Coeli* (IC) – at exact opposite sides of the Zodiac. There are also the moon nodes, called the *Dragon's Head* and the *Dragon's Tail*, exactly opposite one another in the horoscope.

Since the above components are all dealt with similarly in astrology and the horoscope, I allow myself to group them as planets.

Some astrologers include additional points and celestial bodies, but the twelve most important planets and the characters of their forces are:

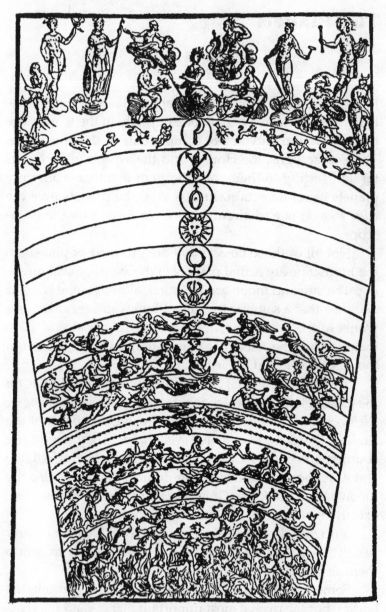

The ancient universe, from the realm of the dead at the bottom to that of the gods at the top. From Cataris, Immagini degli antichi, 1605.

Planet		Force
☉	Sun	basic drive
☽	Moon	longing
☿	Mercury	curiosity
♀	Venus	affection
♂	Mars	aggression
♃	Jupiter	luck
♄	Saturn	duty
♅	Uranus	contemplation
♆	Neptune	fantasy
♇	Pluto	catharsis
AC	Ascendant (AC)	attitude
MC	Medium Coeli (MC)	self-image

Velocity

Some of the above move as fast as one full rotation around the Zodiac in a day, and the slowest one needs almost 250 years to do the same. This is important to consider in the interpretation of a horoscope. The positions of the slower planets are shared almost by a whole generation of people, which is why they are called generation planets. The quicker ones can be said to be more personal, since they move significantly in a matter of days or less.

Here are the times it takes for them to make one rotation around the Zodiac, in round numbers – from a geocentric perspective, i.e. as seen from Earth.

Planet	Orbit
Sun	1 year
Moon	1 month
Mercury	1 year
Venus	1 year
Mars	2 years
Jupiter	12 years

Saturn	29 years
Uranus	84 years
Neptune	164 years
Pluto	248 years
Ascendant (AC)	1 day
Medium Coeli (MC)	1 day

When interpreting a generation planet in the horo-scope, what House it occupies is more important than its Zodiac sign, since the latter is shared by all people born around that time.

Retrograde   ℞
Because the perspective in astrology is geocentric – seen from earth – planets do at times seem to move backwards in the sky. This movement is called *retrograde*, and is the result of earth's own movement. In the horoscope, planets that are in retrograde are marked out as such, since this is taken into consideration in the interpretation of the horoscope.

Generally speaking, retrograde planets are weakened and their force becomes more subtle and diffuse.

Astrological characters
In the actual sky more than in the horoscope, the sun and moon stand out from the other planets. But in astrology all planets are significant and active in their separate ways – not at all shaded by the sun and moon the way they are in the sky to the naked eye.

How the planets were given their respective astrologi-cal characters (as listed above) is buried in the past. Any astrologer would like to regard it as a development of trial and error: Experience taught astrology the meanings of the planets.

Seven of the planets are visible to the naked eye – the

sun, the moon, Mercury, Venus, Mars, Jupiter and Saturn. The outer planets were only discovered after the invention of the telescope, and quite late at that – Uranus in the 18th century, Neptune in the 19th and Pluto in the 20th. The meanings of these planets in the horoscope have largely been deducted from the characteristics of the times of their discovery.

Rulers

Planets are traditionally said to rule over Zodiac signs, in which they are enforced by the character the sign gives them. A planet rules over the Zodiac sign where it fits better than other planets do. It should not be stressed too much in horoscope interpretation, since that enforcement is evident in itself, when the planet's kind of force and the Zodiac sign's character are combined.

Only true celestial bodies can be rulers of Zodiac signs. Since there are just ten of them, and the Zodiac contains twelve signs, two planets rule two signs each. Astrologers agree on most, but not all, of the rulers. Here are the planets and the signs where I would say they rule:

Planet	Ruling sign
Sun	Leo
Moon	Cancer
Mercury	Gemini and Virgo
Venus	Taurus and Libra
Mars	Aries
Jupiter	Sagittarius
Saturn	Capricorn
Uranus	Aquarius
Neptune	Pisces
Pluto	Scorpio

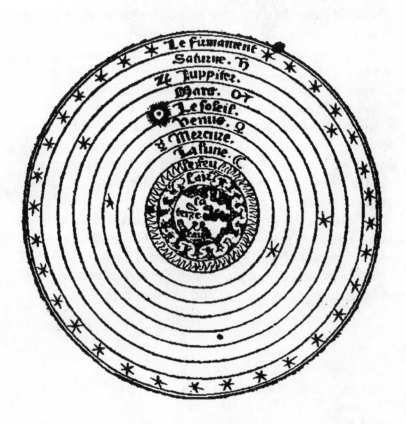

The heavenly spheres. Illustration from a 16th century book by Bovillus (Charles de Bouelles). The Earth is in the center. The closest heavenly body is the moon, next Mercury and Venus, followed by the sun, Mars, Jupiter, and Saturn. The order is that of their velocity through the Zodiac, as seen from Earth. The outmost sphere is that of the Firmament, with the stars. In the days of Bovillus, the outer planets were yet to be discovered.

Your Health in Your Horoscope

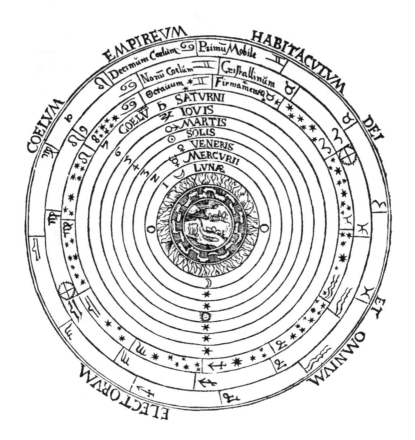

Another illustration of the heavenly spheres, from Cosmographia by Peter Apian, 1540. It also specifies the constellations as well as the even division of heaven into twelve Zodiac signs.

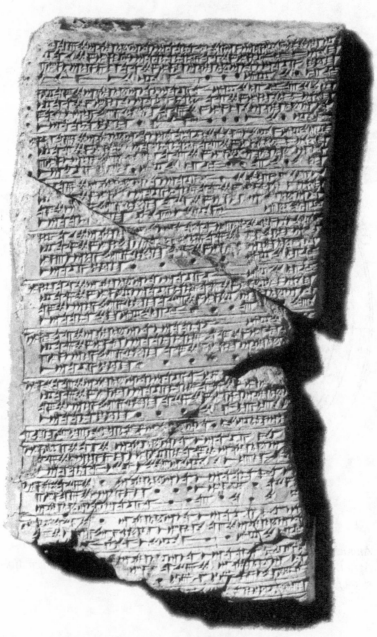

Babylonian clay tablet listing the positions of Venus, circa 700 BC.

Your Health in Your Horoscope

Exalting

The planets are also said to exalt in Zodiac signs – that is where they are enforced, but not to the extent they are in the signs they rule. Again, this should not be overly emphasized in horoscope reading, and again astrologers are of slightly differing opinions. Here are the signs in which I would say the planets exalt:

Planet	Exalting sign
Sun	Aries
Moon	Taurus
Mercury	Libra and Pisces
Venus	Cancer and Virgo
Mars	Capricorn
Jupiter	Gemini
Saturn	Aquarius
Uranus	Sagittarius
Neptune	Scorpio
Pluto	Leo

Symbols

The symbols used for the planets are the same in astrology and astronomy. Here is a strict rendering of them:

⊙ ☽ ☿ ♀ ♂ ♃ ♄ ♅ ♆ ♇ AC MC ☊

Planet symbols. From left to right: Sun, moon, Mercury, Venus, Mars, Jupiter, Saturn, Uranus, Neptune, Pluto, Ascendant, Medium Coeli, moon node.

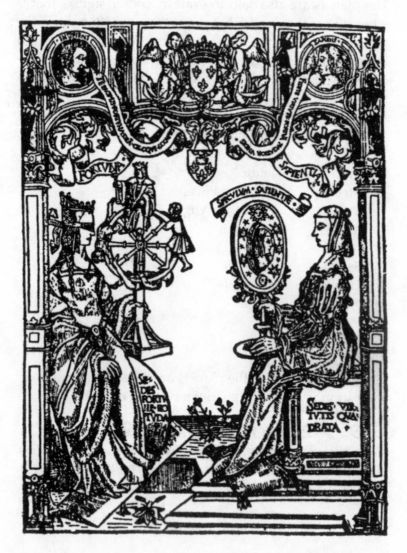

Fortuna and Sapienta. The former, sitting to the left, is here represent-
ing chance and superstition, whereas the latter, to the right, stands for
knowledge and wisdom. Allegoric illustration from Liber de sapiente by
Bovillus (Charles de Bouelles), 1510.

The Houses

In the horoscope chart, the twelve Houses are environments, fields in life where planetary energies are expressed, according to those planets and the tendency given to them by the Zodiac sign they are in. In that way, the Houses give the *where* to events and circumstances indicated by the horoscope.

Here are the twelve Houses, and keywords for what part of life they describe:

House	Keyword
1st House	*Identity*. How others see you.
2nd House	*Resources*. Your personal ability and economy.
3rd House	*Communication*. Your friends and acquaintances, also education.
4th House	*Home*. Your home and family.
5th House	*Pastime*. Your personal preferences, pleasures and interests.
6th House	*Work*. Your profession and daily work.
7th House	*Partners*. Your partners in love and other relations.
8th House	*Unknown*. What you cannot control – fate as well as bloodline.
9th House	*Travel*. Changes of your perspective.
10th House	*Career*. Your social status.
11th House	*Ideals*. Your ideals, and your interaction in the community.
12th House	*Shortcomings*. Your sacrifices, what you are unable to express.

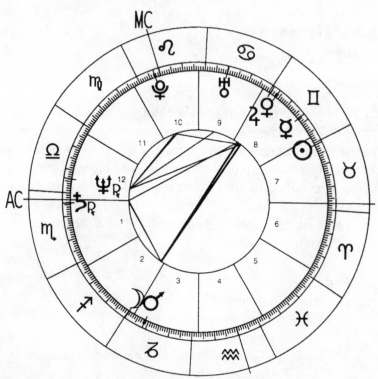

A horoscope chart with the numbered Houses like pizza slices inside the
Zodiac circle. Here are the 12 Houses and their keywords:

1st House	Identity
2nd House	Resources
3rd House	Communication
4th House	Home
5th House	Pastime
6th House	Work
7th House	Partners
8th House	Unknown
9th House	Travel
10th House	Career
11th House	Ideals
12th House	Shortcomings

Zodiac mirror

The Houses are sort of mirrors of the twelve Zodiac signs, so that the part of life each House concerns is deducted from the characteristics of its corresponding Zodiac sign:

House	Sign
1st House	Aries
2nd House	Taurus
3rd House	Gemini
4th House	Cancer
5th House	Leo
6th House	Virgo
7th House	Libra
8th House	Scorpio
9th House	Sagittarius
10th House	Capricorn
11th House	Aquarius
12th House	Pisces

In the horoscope chart, the House system spins around the Zodiac counterclockwise. What decides the House positions is the Ascendant (AC), the Rising point in the east. That's the cusp of the 1st House. The Ascendant travels a full 360° through the Zodiac each day, so it can be in any position in the Zodiac. The rest of the Houses follow in strict order.

Because of the fast movement of the Ascendant through the Zodiac, the House positions can differ considerably even for people born at almost the same time. In the horoscopes of twins the House positions are just about the only significant differences.

House systems

There are several ways of calculating the House positions. The most established ones in western astrology are *Placidus* and *Equal House*.

In the former, Houses have differing sizes, and *Medium Coeli* (MC) is at the cusp of the 10th House. Also, the *Descendant* starts the 7th House, and the *Imum Coeli* (IC) starts the 4th House. In the latter, all Houses are of the same 30° size, as its name suggests. The MC can be anywhere from House 7 to 12, but the Ascendant is always at the cusp of the 1st House, and the Descendant at that of the 7th House.

I prefer the Equal House system for several reasons. It matches the sizes of the Zodiac signs, which are equal, and it is the oldest system, supported already by Ptolemy. Furthermore, it keeps the aspecting relations between the Houses intact – a relation that helps a lot in understanding the Houses and interpreting them in the chart.

Aspects between Houses

A good example of the aspect relations between the Houses is the *opposition*, 180° apart. This aspect points out irreconcilable differences, opposing interests or perspectives that usually relate only as "either or".

These are the oppositions of the Houses:

Houses in opposition
1st – 7th House
2nd – 8th House
3rd – 9th House
4th – 10th House
5th – 11th House
6th – 12th House

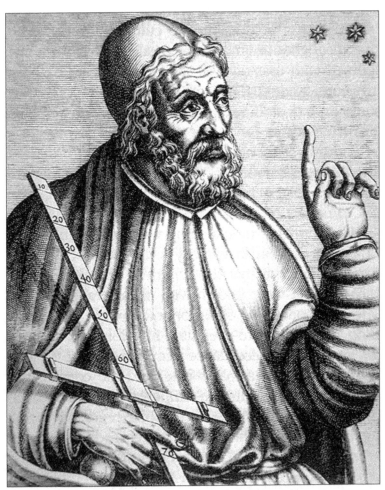

Ptolemy (c. 85-168 CE), Greek astronomer and mathematician. He wrote Tetrabiblos, a book about astrology that is still the basic source of European astrology. This Renaissance portrait by an unknown artist is made with no knowledge of what Ptolemy actually looked like.

Introduction to Medical Astrology

The opposition is very clear and indisputable in many of the above – such as between one's home and one's career (4th and 10th) or one's personal interests and one's ideals (5th and 11th).

The opposition is present also in non-Equal House systems, since opposing Houses are the same size also there, but that is not necessarily the case with other aspects.

The *trine* (120°) points out harmonious relations, things that work in accordance with each other. Here are the trines of the Houses, which correspond to Zodiac signs of the same element:

Houses in trine	Element
1st – 5th – 9th House	fire
2nd – 6th – 10th House	earth
3rd – 7th – 11th House	air
4th – 8th – 12th House	water

The element fire signifies activity, earth signifies material matters, air thought, and water emotions. What each House signifies has a lot to do with these elemental characters. Thus, the earth Houses deal with material things, the water Houses with emotions, and so on.

The *square* (90°) points out conflicts, things that work against each other – either in a productive or a destructive way. In the Zodiac, signs at square distance have the same quality – cardinal, fixed or mutable.

Here are the House squares:

Houses in square	Quality
1st – 4th – 7th – 10th House	cardinal
2nd – 5th – 8th – 11th House	fixed
3rd – 6th – 9th – 12th House	mutable

The cardinal is the leading, the fixed is unwilling to change at all, and the mutable is the following. The Houses can be described accordingly.

Finally, the *sextile* (60°) describes cooperation, things that work well together. In the Zodiac this corresponds to signs that are said to have either a positive or a negative charge. Fire and air signs are regarded as positive, while earth and water signs are negative. Thus, in the Zodiac circle, every other sign is positive and every other negative. Here are the House sextiles:

Houses in sextile	Charge
1st – 3rd – 5th – 7th – 9th – 11th House	positive
2nd – 4th – 6th – 8th – 10th – 12th House	negative

There's no preference or evaluation implied by the words positive and negative. Rather, they are to be regarded as complementary, sort of like the Chinese idea of yin-yang. Positive is expansive, negative is contracting. The Houses also show these tendencies.

Environment

So, much of the significance of each House can be told by the characteristics described above, shown by the aspects and the Zodiac signs to which they correspond. Still, it must be remembered that the Houses do not equal the Zodiac signs. They just carry their traits in the environment or part of life they relate to. Here are all the above Zodiac traits for each House:

HOUSE	Zodiac sign	Element - quality - charge
1st House	Aries	fire – cardinal – positive
2nd House	Taurus	earth – fixed – negative
3rd House	Gemini	air – mutable – positive

4th House	Cancer	water – cardinal – negative
5th House	Leo	fire – fixed – positive
6th House	Virgo	earth – mutable – negative
7th House	Libra	air – cardinal – positive
8th House	Scorpio	water – fixed – negative
9th House	Sagittarius	fire – mutable – positive
10th House	Capricorn	earth – cardinal – negative
11th House	Aquarius	air – fixed – positive
12th House	Pisces	water – mutable – negative

House positions

Remember that in the horoscope chart, the Houses can be in any other signs than those they have gotten much of their characteristics from. The 1st House can be in Aries, but also in any other sign of the Zodiac. The rest of the Houses follow in strict order, so a certain position of the Ascendant (AC) leads to the Houses arranging themselves accordingly.

One might presume that if the Houses are indeed in their "natural" signs – the 1st in Aries and so on – it would be the most agreeable position, but that is not necessarily so. When Houses and Zodiac signs match that well, it can tend to dim the dynamics of the chart, so that things get a bit too predictable, too typical, with little room for originality and surprise.

Already if the Houses are in signs of opposite charge – positive in negative, and vice versa – this stimulates and gives ground for creativity. In opposing signs there is a chance to accomplish balance in one's life, in trine signs different aspects of life can run quite smoothly, whereas in square signs it can either be very constructive or a complete mess. The unique mix of the ingredients in a chart shows personality, and that's what makes life an intriguing challenge.

Your Health in Your Horoscope

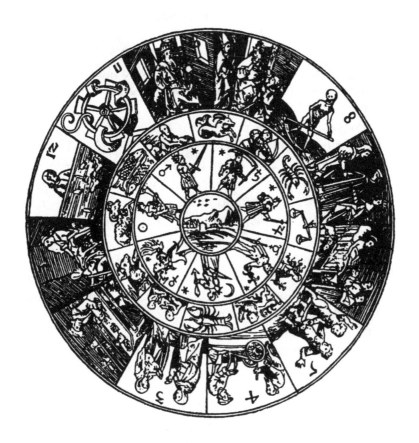

The Houses of the horoscope, from a book by the astronomer Georg von Peuerbach (1423-1461). The illustration shows the links between the planets, the Zodiac signs, and the astrological Houses. The images in the Houses indicate the parts of life they represent.

Introduction to Medical Astrology

Split sign

Usually, the Houses are split between two signs. Rarely are the cusps of the Houses exactly at the cusps of the Zodiac signs. This must be taken into account in the interpretation of the horoscope.

There are two major considerations needed – that of time and that of dominance.

Time works so that the environment of a House will at first have the character of the first sign, and later that of the next sign. Their extension in time will be comparable to the share the signs have of the House.

For example, if the 6th House is one third Pisces and two thirds Aries, then that person's work will at first be a bit confused, searching for a way to do it right, and then active, intense, maybe rushing it. Each new work the person gets will follow this pattern, and in the same proportions – one third of the employment according to the first sign, the rest according to the following sign.

Dominance is something less precise. If most of a House is in one sign, that sign's character will have a tendency to dominate, through all time. Even more so if there are planets in one sign and not in the other. The positions of the planets are the most important when interpreting how things will be in the environment that the House describes.

Empty Houses

Houses void of planets mark fields of life where not that much happens, at least not very significant things. Those environments are not the most important ones in that person's life.

The Aspects

In the horoscope chart, the aspects are certain angles between planets or astrological points in the chart. The aspects
show how these points relate and interact. In that way, the
aspects give the *why* to events and circumstances indicated
by the horoscope.

When a chart is interpreted, the aspects bring it all together and turn the symbols of the diagram into a complete
human being.

These are the major aspects in astrology:

Aspect		Angle
♂	Conjunction	0°
☍	Opposition	180°
△	Trine	120°
□	Square	90°
✶	Sextile	60°

Some astrologers use additional aspects, such as the
quincunx (150°) and the *semisextile* (30°), but the above are
the most important ones. They are also the ones specified by
Ptolemy in his classic on astrology, *Tetrabiblos*. I prefer to
stick to these five aspects – they sure make the horoscope
chart complex enough.

Each aspect represents a kind of relation between the
planets or astrological points connected by it:

Aspect	Effect
conjunction, 0°	blending
opposition, 180°	separation

trine, 120°	harmony
square, 90°	conflict
sextile, 60°	cooperation

Order of importance

The strongest aspect is the *conjunction*, where planets or astrological points are very near each other in the chart. The blending means that they become like one, their separate characters melting into one, like a new planet. You could also call it a synthesis of the forces involved.

Second in power is the *opposition*, where the planets are on opposite sides of the chart. This signifies that the forces of those planets are irreconcilable, impossible to get to work together. They get a relation of "either-or", so that either one or the other planet acts – but not simultaneously, never joined.

Third in power is the *trine*, which shows harmony between the planets at that angle. Their forces work for one another, not necessarily through actual cooperation, but still being mutually helpful.

Fourth in power is the *square*, which reveals complications between the planets involved – conflicting interests that can either be constructive or destructive.

The weakest of these five aspects is the *sextile*, showing active cooperation, where the planets involved concretely aid one another and work together.

Orb

Astrologers differ as to how exact the angles should be in order to be called aspects. The tolerance given is called *orb*. With an orb of 5°, anything from 85° to 95° would be a square, and so on. Some use orbs as big as 10°, but I prefer to use narrow orbs, in order for the chart to really point out strong and relevant aspects. An orb of 4° would do fine.

Your Health in Your Horoscope

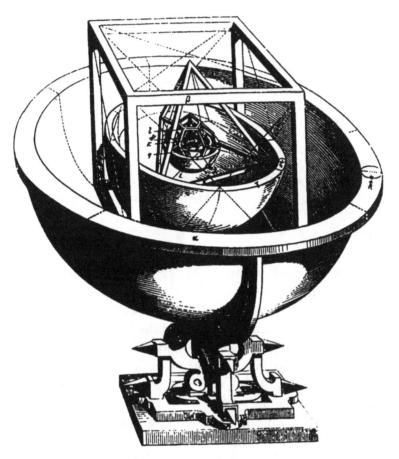

Johannes Kepler's model for the solar system, with the planets at distances from the sun that correspond to geometric figures. Kepler (1571-1630) was a mathematician and astronomer, but also an astrologer. In his astrological interpretations he put great emphasis on the aspects and their harmonies (using the numbers by which they divide the full Zodiac circle). His way of reasoning about this was in line with what is called the Music of the Spheres. The illustration is from his book Mysterium Cosmographicum, 1621.

Another solution is to use different orbs for each aspect, in accordance with their strength and importance. Then, something like this would be reasonable:

Aspect	Orb
conjunction, 0°	5° orb, 0°-5°
opposition, 180°	5° orb, 175°-180°
trine, 120°	4° orb, 116°-124°
square, 90°	3° orb, 87°-93°
sextile, 60°	2° orb, 58°-62°

Notice that the trine, square and sextile can appear on both sides of a planet. For example, the sun in Leo can make a trine to either a planet in Aries or one in Sagittarius.

Origin

The conjunction and the opposition are obvious aspects, but how about the other three? They are connected to relations within the Zodiac circle.

The twelve signs of the Zodiac are sorted in three ways: *element*, *quality* and *charge*. Signs of the same element (fire, earth, air or water) are 120° apart, like the trine. Signs of the same quality (cardinal, fixed or mutable) are 90° apart, like the square. Signs of the same charge (positive or negative) are 60° apart, like the sextile.

Another likely influence in the forming of the classic aspects is quite likely to be mathematical. The 360° of the circle divided by 2 is 180°, the opposition, with 3 is 120°, the trine, with 4 is 90°, the square, and with 6 is 60°, the sextile. Division by 5 gives 72°, which is also an aspect, called the *quintile*, but it is not regarded as particularly significant.

Aspects can appear between two planets that are not in the corresponding aspected Zodiac signs, because of the orb allowed. For example, if the sun is in 1° Aries and the moon

Your Health in Your Horoscope

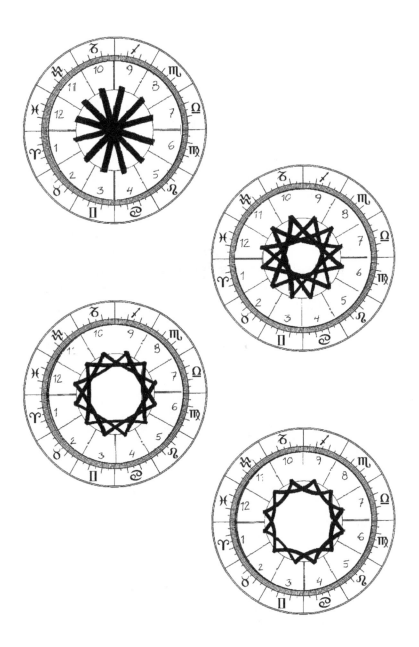

The aspects and their relations to the Zodiac signs and the Houses. From top to bottom: opposition, trine, square, and sextile.

Introduction to Medical Astrology

is in 29° Pisces, they are only at a 2° distance, although in separate signs – so, do they still form a conjunction? They do, but the interpretation of what kind of fusion it is must take into account what characteristics they get from their separate signs. There are four ingredients to mix in such a case.

I would say that in this way an aspect "over the border" is weaker and more subtle than one where the planets are in aspected Zodiac signs as well.

Velocity

When interpreting birth charts, it's important to remember that aspects remain for very different time periods, because of the differing speeds of the planets in their orbits. Here is the time it takes each planet to travel through the whole Zodiac:

Planet	Orbit
Sun	1 year
Moon	1 month
Mercury	1 year
Venus	1 year
Mars	2 years
Jupiter	12 years
Saturn	29 years
Uranus	84 years
Neptune	164 years
Pluto	248 years

Depending on the orb allowed, an aspect between Neptune and Pluto can last for years, even decades, whereas one with the moon can disappear in mere hours. Very slow aspects are shared by whole generations, and should be interpreted accordingly. With those it is more important in

Your Health in Your Horoscope

what Houses they are, than what Zodiac signs they occupy. Also, of course, other faster aspects with them should be given special attention.

The most rare aspects are the conjunction and opposition of Neptune and Pluto, appearing only every 487 years. Last time they formed such an aspect was their conjunction around the year 1892 at about 8° Gemini.

Special cases

You should know that the mean positions of the AC and MC are at square distance – more so, the closer you get to the equator. Trines between them are quite rare, and oppositions are almost impossible.

About Mercury and Venus you should know that they never get that far from the sun, in the geocentric perspective of the horoscope. They can only form a conjunction with the sun, and nothing but a conjunction or a sextile with one another. Mercury is never more than 28° from the sun, Venus never more than 38°.

Progressions and transits

Aspects are also the major instruments in making predictions based on the horoscope chart. It is done by *progression* and *transit*.

In *progression*, what is observed is a theoretical (not actual) advance of the planets in the horoscope chart, until they form aspects with other planets or astrological points in it. The distance traveled equals a certain time gone until that event.

In *transit*, the actual continued movements of the planets are observed. The date when a new aspect is formed with a planet in the birth chart is the time for an event characterized by the involved planets.

I prefer the transit predictions, since the progressions

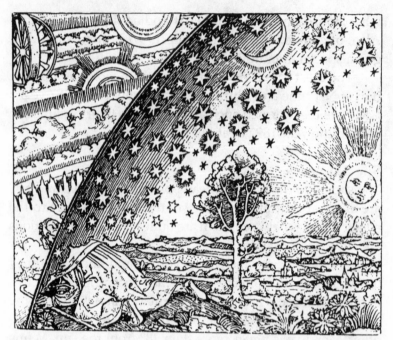

The Medieval world. Woodprint by Camille Flammarion 1888, often mistakenly believed to be a picture from the Renaissance era.

are more difficult to find solid arguments for. When you use the transits, remember that rare aspects are much more important than frequent ones. So, aspects with the transit moon accomplish little more than mood swings, whereas aspects with transit Pluto are likely to change your whole life from that moment on.

Symbols

The symbols used for the aspects are the same in astrology and astronomy. Here is a strict rendering of them:

☌ ☍ △ □ ✳

Aspect symbols: conjunction, opposition, trine, square, sextile.

Your health in
your horoscope

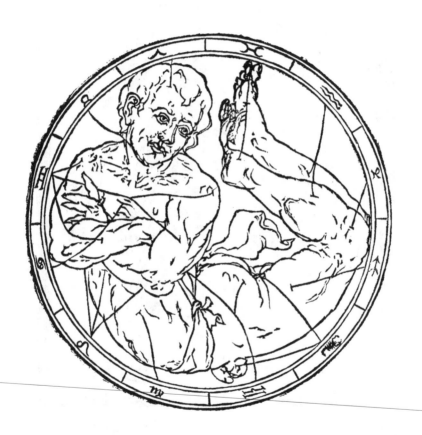

*Zodiac Man. Illustration from Margarita Philosophicae by Gregorius
Reisch, 1599.*

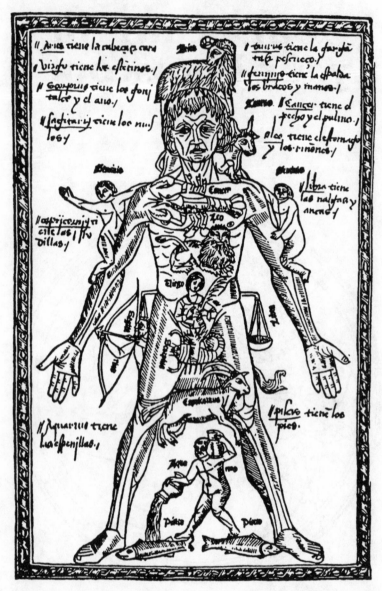

Zodiac Man, a common motif in the history of astrology, showing what body parts the Zodiac signs govern. Traditionally, this was done from Aries for the head to Pisces for the feet, like in this Medieval illustration.

Your Health in Your Horoscope

Your health in your horoscope

Since ancient times, astrology has been used also to track health problems and find ways to solve them. It is usually called medical astrology, or with a traditional term *Iatro-mathematics* (the math of curing). Your horoscope gives several clues to your health and what you might do to improve problems you may have with it.

There are four major factors at work in the horoscope, also when it comes to health indicators:

1   what
2   how
3   where
4   why

In the horoscope, each one of those four ingredients is represented by one of its four components:

1   *Planets* and similar points in the horoscope show *what* happens, what active power is at work.
2   *Zodiac* signs show *how* the planets act, the characteristics of the event.
3   *Houses* show *where* in one's life, in what environment, the planets act.
4   *Aspects*, the special angles between planets, show *why* the planets act as they do.

It's the same regarding your health. An obstructed planet can cause health problems linked to its own nature, and with the characteristics of the Zodiac sign the planet is

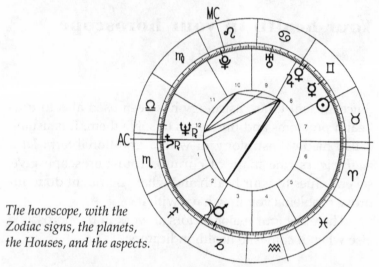

The horoscope, with the Zodiac signs, the planets, the Houses, and the aspects.

in. Usually it strikes the body part governed by that Zodiac sign. Your health problem will be particularly influential and apparent in the environment of the House the planet is in. The reason for the planet causing trouble is seen in the aspects it forms to other planets – either those of your birth chart, or planets in the sky that form transit aspects to those in your chart.

That's really all you need to examine. But of course, it takes some time to sort out and understand these variables correctly.

A good way to familiarize yourself with how your horoscope indicates your health problems is to analyze illnesses or other health issues in your past. See if you can explain them by your birth chart, or by transits at play at the time of those ailments.

You will have to choose significant health problems that you may have had, in order to find clear indicators of them in your horoscope. Not just any cold.

Study your past to know your future. That's as true for astrology as it is for life in general.

Your Health in Your Horoscope

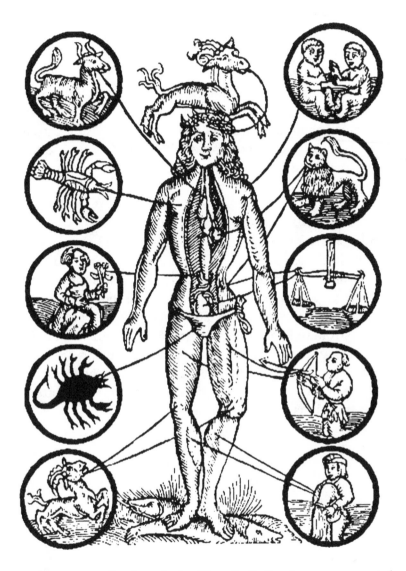

Zodiac Man. Medieval woodprint. Here, the Zodiac signs are represented by pictures instead of the traditional symbols. This is also common through astrological history. Aries is at the top of the man's head, and Pisces below his feet. The other signs are to the sides.

Introduction to Medical Astrology   67

The Zodiac and your health

Only the planets and astrological points are the active forces in your horoscope. But the Zodiac signs they occupy will tell you much about the nature of their actions, also in regard to your health. The planets cause illnesses, but the Zodiac signs reveal the nature of those illnesses and the body parts afflicted by them.

Zodiac Man

Traditionally, the twelve Zodiac signs are said to represent twelve body parts, from the head down. It's referred to as the *Zodiac Man*, or *Astrological Man*, who is a common motif in illustrations of the Middle Ages and the Renaissance. You see several examples of such images in this book.

Astrology is not in total agreement about what body part belongs to what sign, but the pattern is mainly the same – from Aries and the head down to Pisces and the feet. Here is a list of the Zodiac signs and the body parts they are in most traditions said to be connected to:

Sign	Body part
Aries	head
Taurus	neck, throat, ears
Gemini	lungs, arms, fingers
Cancer	chest
Leo	heart, blood
Virgo	abdomen
Libra	hips, kidneys
Scorpio	genitals, rectum
Sagittarius	thighs

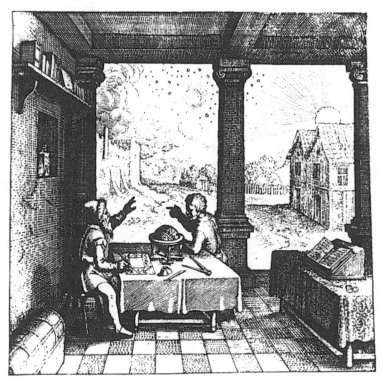
Astrologers at work. Renaissance woodprint.

Capricorn	knees
Aquarius	ankles
Pisces	feet

The Zodiac is very helpful in astrological diagnosis, but the meaning of each sign needs to be modified somewhat. On the following pages, I suggest how they should be interpreted in the horoscope, from applying astrological principles to their roles in the body.

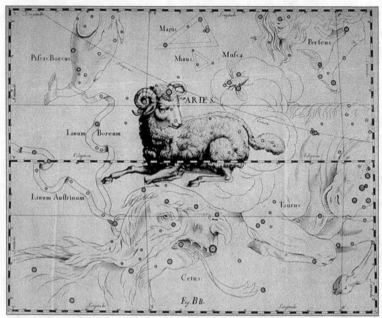

Aries, the constellation. Illustration from Firmamentum sobiescianum, by Johannes Hevelius, 1690.

♈

Aries

Aries governs the head and brain, and their ailments – damages to the skull as well as headaches and brain hemorrhage. Aries is the sign of challenge and impatience, so a high tempo and restless excitement is likely to lead to problems of the head. Stress is the most obvious example, leading to migraine and even to brain hemorrhage. On the other hand, people who have Aries strengthened by planets in the sign can take a lot of heat.

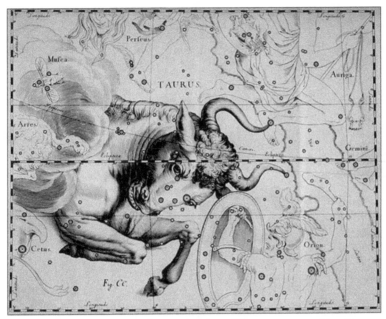

Taurus, the constellation. Illustration from Firmamentum sobiescianum, by Johannes Hevelius, 1690.

Taurus

Taurus governs the throat, neck and ears, also the nose, teeth, and hearing. A strong Taurus gives good hearing and fine teeth, but still an openness to flu and the common cold. A weakened Taurus easily results in getting a cold or a flu, also hoarseness and problems with the teeth.

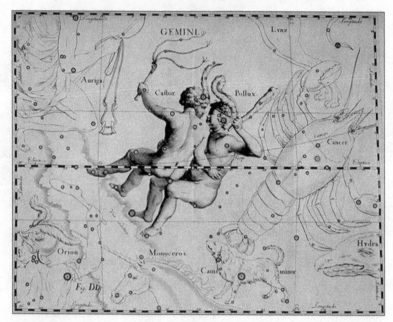

Gemini, the constellation. Illustration from Firmamentum sobiescianum, by Johannes Hevelius, 1690.

♊

Gemini

Gemini governs speech, smell, and the lungs – all things dependent on the flow of air in breathing. Therefore, a strong as well as a weakened Gemini tends to attract the common cold, whereas a weakened Gemini is also sensitive to flu and cough. Asthma and other complications of the breath are also connected to Gemini.

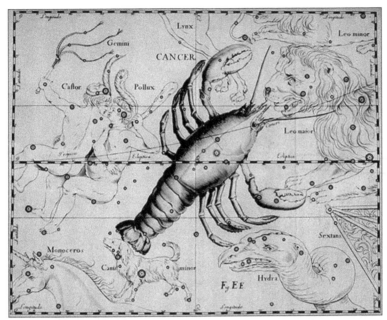

Cancer, the constellation. Illustration from Firmamentum sobiescianum, by Johannes Hevelius, 1690.

Cancer

Cancer governs the skin, which is the organ for the sense of touch. A weakened Cancer creates skin problems of all kinds. Also a strong Cancer is open to some skin ailments – but it usually results in very healthy skin, sometimes almost radiant.

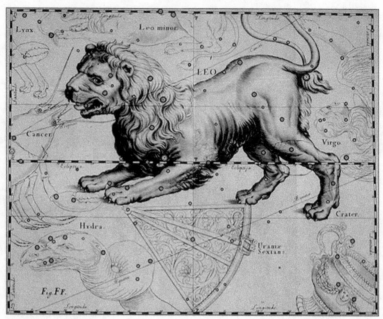

Leo, the constellation. Illustration from Firmamentum sobiescianum, by Johannes Hevelius, 1690.

Leo

Leo governs the heart and the blood. A weakened Leo influences the heart beat and how the blood flows in one's body, which is cause for concern. A strengthened Leo makes the heart sturdy and the blood healthy – up to a point. Beyond that point there is a risk of high blood pressure and exhaustion of the heart.

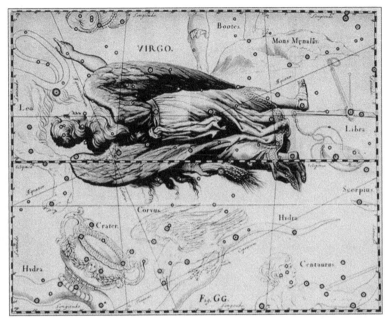

Virgo, the constellation. Illustration from Firmamentum sobiescianum, by Johannes Hevelius, 1690.

Virgo

Virgo governs the food intake and related intestines, especially the stomach. A weakened Virgo leads to eating disorders and stomach ache. Those with a strengthened Virgo can eat just about anything. Ulcer and other stomach ailments are usually connected to Virgo in some way.

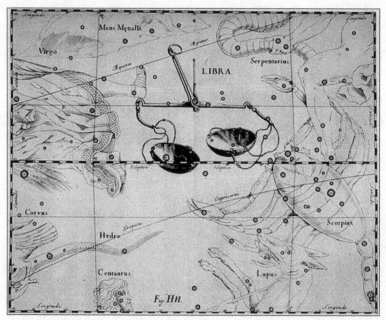

Libra, the constellation. Illustration from Firmamentum sobiescianum, by Johannes Hevelius, 1690.

Libra

Libra governs the food processing intestines that absorb nutrition, and the excrement. A weakened Libra results in digestion problems, also things like constipation or the opposite. A strong Libra can lead to similar problems, but mostly makes the metabolism run like clockwork.

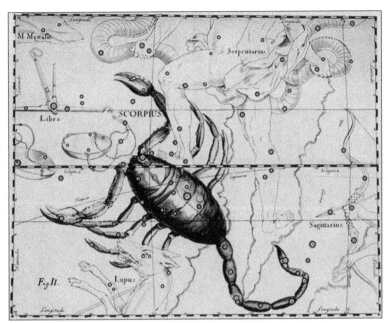

Scorpio, the constellation. Illustration from Firmamentum sobiescianum, *by Johannes Hevelius, 1690.*

Scorpio

Scorpio governs the genitals and the hormones. A weakened Scorpio can lead to diminished sex drive, and a strengthened Scorpio to the opposite. Venereal disease is very much related to Scorpio, and so is the urine. The effects on the hormones are usually subtle and difficult to observe – but they can certainly get devastating.

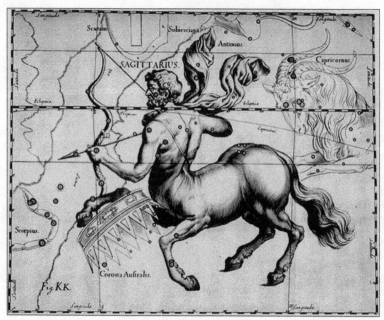

*Sagittarius, the constellation. Illustration from Firmamentum sobiescia-
num, by Johannes Hevelius, 1690.*

Sagittarius

Sagittarius governs the eyes and eyesight. A weakened
Sagittarius leads to impaired vision, whereas a strengthened
Sagittarius is likely to give perfect eyesight, especially at a
distance.

Your Health in Your Horoscope

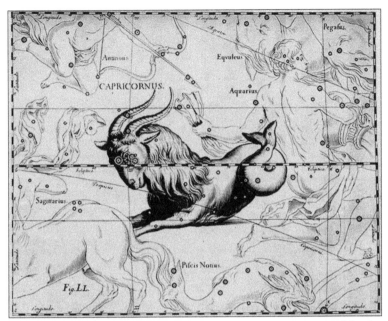

*Capricorn, the constellation. Illustration from Firmamentum sobiescia-
num, by Johannes Hevelius, 1690.*

♑

Capricorn

Capricorn governs the bones of the body. They are strong if
Capricorn is, and weak when Capricorn is. Accidents in-
volving the bones can be spotted in Capricorn. Especially
the spine is a Capricorn thing, therefore also one's posture.

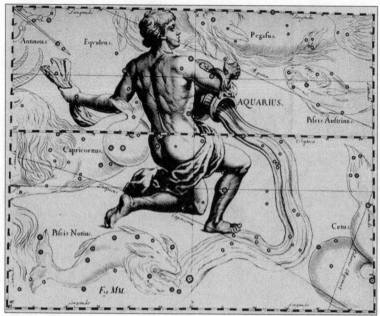

Aquarius, the constellation. Illustration from Firmamentum sobiescia-
num, by Johannes Hevelius, 1690.

Aquarius

Aquarius governs the arms and legs, and one's ability to
move about in general. A weakened Aquarius causes impaired movement, for example clumsiness, whereas a
strengthened Aquarius gives stamina and elegance to the
movements. The hands and feet are related to Aquarius, but
they tend also to be influenced by some other signs,
depending on the situation and ailment.

Your Health in Your Horoscope

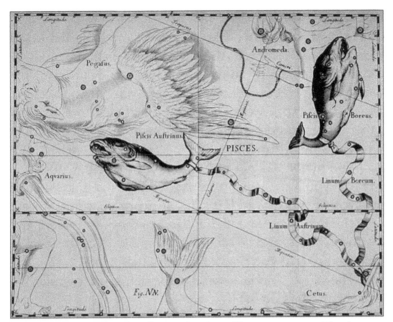

Pisces, the constellation. Illustration from Firmamentum sobiescianum, by Johannes Hevelius, 1690.

Pisces

Pisces governs the nervous system, therefore also the reflexes. A weakened Pisces can lead to erratic behavior and some unintentional body spasms, whereas a strengthened Pisces leads to composition and calmness – up to a point. Several but not all the ailments of the psyche are related to Pisces.

Muscles

Far from all the body parts and organs are included in the lists above. For example, there is no mention of the muscles, although they are certainly essential to survival. That's because they can't be connected to one single Zodiac sign. Muscular qualities vary according to their functions and other things – and planets play a role in their development as well as their durability.

The major but not only planet of muscular power is Mars. If you have Mars in Taurus, you are likely to be quite strong in a sturdy way. If it's in Capricorn your muscles are sufficient and resourceful, if it's in Leo they are evident and impress others, and so on. With Mars in Pisces or Gemini, chances are that you're not that muscular at all.

The sun, too, indicates muscular status, pretty much the same way Mars does.

Power in Zodiac signs

The Zodiac is a background in the horoscope. It doesn't represent actual powers or energies at play. Instead, it gives certain characteristics to them. The working powers in the horoscope are the planets, including the sun and moon, the Ascendant (AC) and Medium Coeli (MC). These are the active ingredients in the horoscope.

A Zodiac sign without any of the planets is not really weakened, from a health perspective. What it implies is that health issues belonging to that Zodiac sign are no real problems. The empty Zodiac signs in your horoscope show that you rarely have ailments in the body parts those signs govern.

There are three exceptions: if a Zodiac sign is in the 12th, 6th or 8th House, it can cause some trouble whether it's empty or not. More about that below, when the roles of the Houses in your health are discussed.

As for Zodiac signs that have planets in your horoscope, it generally means they are enhanced. A planet brings energy to the Zodiac sign, so it becomes stronger and more important – also the body part that it governs.

But there are exceptions to the rule, and several things to consider. A planet in a Zodiac sign can just as well lead to complications. You have to look at the whole picture. Consider aspects, Houses, and where in the Zodiac sign the planet is (see below about decans).

Parts of the Zodiac sign

A Zodiac sign is not exactly the same all through its 30° of the Zodiac circle. The beginning of a sign is forceful, whereas the end of it is kind of dissolving, and there are many nuances in between.

A traditional way of taking this into account is the division of a sign into three parts of 10° each, called *decanate* or *decan*. The first decan is *cardinal* (leading), the middle *fixed*, and the third is *mutable* (following). These three qualitites also sort the Zodiac signs in whole, so that some signs are cardinal, others fixed or mutable.

There is great order to it: Each of the four Greek *elements* (fire, air, earth, and water) have three Zodiac signs, and these three are of one quality each. Here are the elements and qualitites of the Zodiac signs:

Sign	Element	Quality
Aries	fire	cardinal
Taurus	earth	fixed
Gemini	air	mutable
Cancer	water	cardinal
Leo	fire	fixed
Virgo	earth	mutable
Libra	air	cardinal

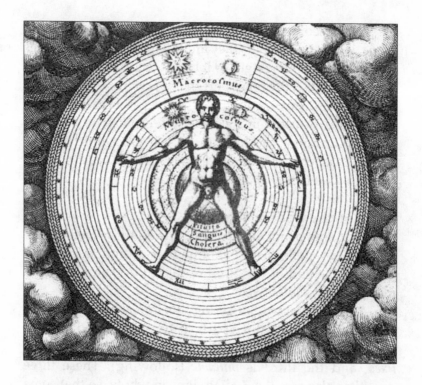

Scorpio	water	fixed
Sagittarius	fire	mutable
Capricorn	earth	cardinal
Aquarius	air	fixed
Pisces	water	mutable

Since a Zodiac sign can also be divided into cardinal, fixed, and mutable decans, a decan of a Zodiac sign tends to be slightly similar to the sign of the same element with the quality of that decan. It also means that a Zodiac sign is the most typical and characteristic in the decan of the quality that the sign itself belongs to.

For example: Aries is the cardinal fire sign, so its first decan, the cardinal one, shows the most distinct Aries traits.

Its second decan, the fixed one, is slightly similar to the fixed fire sign Leo, and its last and mutable decan has some similarities to the mutable fire sign Sagittarius.

Therefore, a Zodiac sign is its strongest in the decan of the quality that the sign belongs to, which is where it is the most characteristic. It is weaker in the other decans. A cardinal sign is at the very weakest, quite frustrated, at its mutable decan, and the other way around. A fixed sign is usually weaker in its mutable decan than in its cardinal decan, but the difference is not that great.

Here are the Zodiac signs, and what other signs they have similarities to in their decans:

Sign	1st decan	2nd decan	3rd decan
Aries	Aries	Leo	Sagittarius
Taurus	Capricorn	Taurus	Virgo
Gemini	Libra	Aquarius	Gemini
Cancer	Cancer	Scorpio	Pisces
Leo	Aries	Leo	Sagittarius
Virgo	Capricorn	Taurus	Virgo
Libra	Libra	Aquarius	Gemini
Scorpio	Cancer	Scorpio	Pisces
Sagittarius	Aries	Leo	Sagittarius
Capricorn	Capricorn	Taurus	Virgo
Aquarius	Libra	Aquarius	Gemini
Pisces	Cancer	Scorpio	Pisces

Regarding your health in your horoscope, you should pay attention to what decan of the Zodiac a planet is in. That tells you a lot about the constitution of that planet, what ailments it might cause, and to what extent.

Each decan of a Zodiac sign tends to narrow down the body part inflicted, or the kind of infliction. It is not that certain or exact, but the table below gives clues to how the

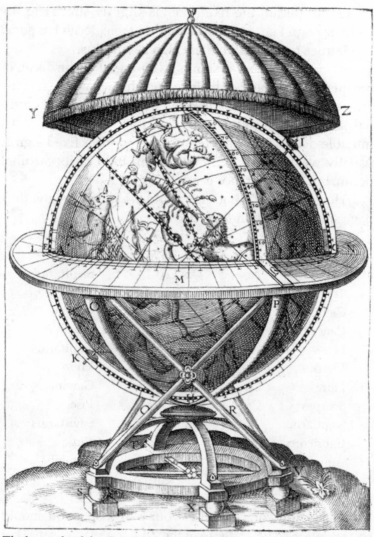

The heavenly globe. From Astronomiae instauratae mechanica by Tycho Brahe, 1602.

decans modify physical ailments and problems of each sign. These are indications, only. Don't take them too literally.

Sign	1st decan	2nd decan	3rd decan
Aries	skull	migraine	concentration
Taurus	nose	throat	ears
Gemini	smell	lungs	speech
Cancer	skin	body fat	touch
Leo	heart	blood	circulation
Virgo	appetite	stomach	digestion
Libra	metabolism	bowels	excrement
Scorpio	sexuality	genitals	hormones
Sagittarius	far-sight	eyes	near-sight
Capricorn	spine	bones	joints
Aquarius	arms	legs	movement
Pisces	coordination	nerves	reflexes

Some Zodiac signs are more prone to cause mental disorders than physical ones. That's even more true about some planets. Still, any mental disorder tends to lead also to some kind of physical malfunction or ailment – and then the above gives a good indication to what.

Planets and your health

While the Zodiac signs govern the body parts than either can be healthy or get struck by illness, the actual forces at play are represented by the planets and astrological points in the horoscope. They are the active parts of the horoscope. The Zodiac and the Houses are their backgrounds. Zodiac signs give character to the planets, and Houses reveal in what environment of your life they are active.

A Zodiac sign with no planet is not very significant, so the body part governed by it is not likely to either excel or cause serious trouble (except for the signs of Houses 12, 6, and 8). If there is a planet in a Zodiac sign, it is enhanced and activated. This normally means increased health, but can sometimes lead to serious problems as well. It depends on the planet and the aspects to it.

Mainly, it depends on how much the force that the planet represents is allowed to act. If its ability is diminished or held back, it sort of retaliates by causing illness or other problems. A planet that can't act according to its positive nature will react in a negative way.

Almost all health problems are caused by planetary powers in the horoscope held back or obstructed.

Each planet has its own way of affecting the health – both in a positive way, when correctly stimulated, and in a negative way when obstructed. Here are the planets and astrological points, and their general effects on your health, when over-stimulated and when obstructed:

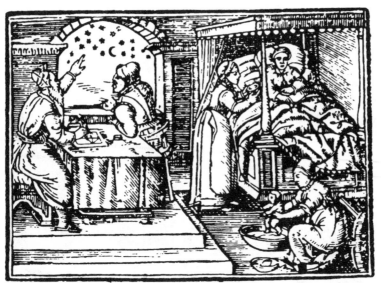

Astrologers observing the stars at a delivery. Renaissance woodprint.

Planet	Over-stimulation	Obstruction
Sun	exertion	fatigue
Moon	desperation	anxiety
Mercury	stress	confusion
Venus	discomfort	dissatisfaction
Mars	strain	pain
Jupiter	exaggeration	misfortune
Saturn	burden	disappointment
Uranus	bewilderment	mistake
Neptune	distraction	boredom
Pluto	destruction	complication
Ascendant	pompousness	unattractiveness
Medium Coeli	self-indulgence	misunderstanding

On the following pages, the planets and their potential health effects are explained in more detail.

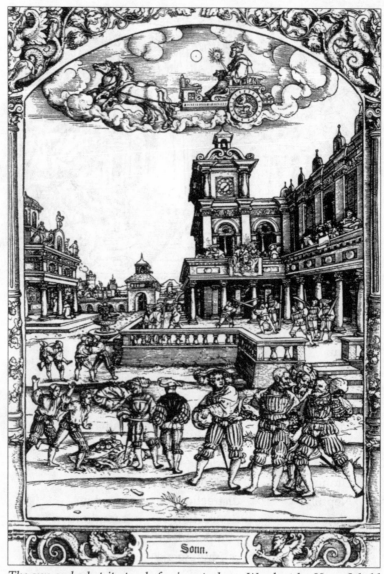

The sun and what it stands for in astrology. Woodcut by Hans Sebald Beham from the 1530's.

Your Health in Your Horoscope

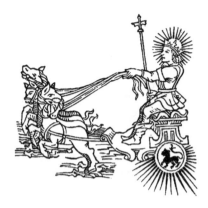

Sun

The sun causes general fatigue and weakness when obstructed, especially but not only in the body part of the Zodiac sign it occupies. On the other hand, when the sun is stimulated or enhanced in some way, it leads to strength and endurance – not only in the body part of its Zodiac sign. Because the sun is a general resource of the horoscope, its health influence is quite general, affecting your well-being more than specific organs.

It is almost impossible to over-stimulate the sun, but when it happens, you might become complacent, even lazy, losing interest in the world around you. It can also unbalance your body by bringing too much power to the body part of the Zodiac sign the sun occupies.

The sun is not particularly weakened in any Zodiac sign, except maybe to a minor degree in Pisces. It is particularly strong – and demanding – in Leo and Aries, also in Capricorn and to some extent in Libra.

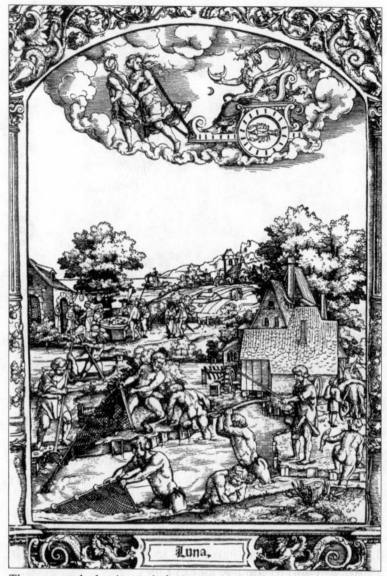

The moon and what it stands for in astrology. Woodcut by Hans Sebald Beham from the 1530's.

Your Health in Your Horoscope

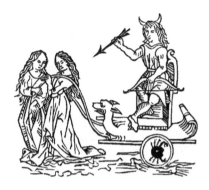

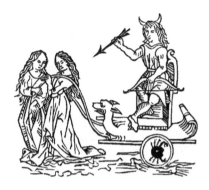

Moon

The moon creates sadness and gloom when obstructed or held back. You can experience a lack of fulfillment that might lead to depression. At length it may also lead to imbalance in bodily fluids. Like the sun, the moon does not only affect the body part of the Zodiac sign it occupies, but your general well-being – especially in regard to your emotions.

When the moon is enhanced and stimulated, it leads to patience, a strong sense of fulfillment, and a persistently good mood. An over-stimulated moon leads to sentimentality, maybe even manic depression outbursts, and a loss of touch with the world.

The moon is somewhat weakened in Virgo and Capricorn, sometimes also in Gemini. It is particularly strong and demanding in Cancer, also in Taurus, Pisces, and Scorpio.

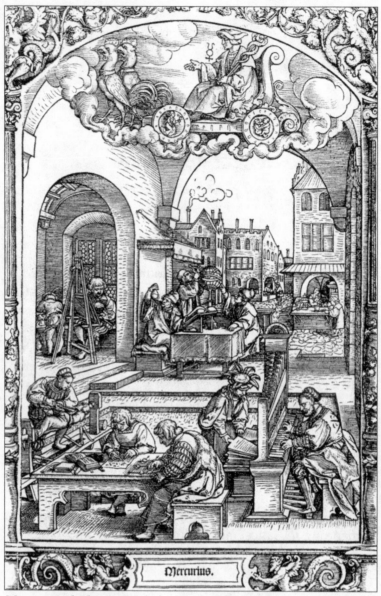

Mercury and what it stands for in astrology. Woodcut by Hans Sebald Beham from the 1530's.

Your Health in Your Horoscope

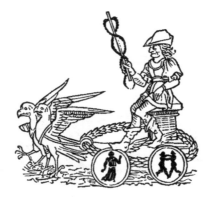

Mercury

Mercury creates nervousness and erratic behavior when obstructed. You may get some spasms in your motions, and have trouble to express yourself or to make your conscious mind work as quickly and smoothly as you expect it to. The planet deals mainly with mental things, whatever Zodiac sign it occupies.

When Mercury is enhanced and stimulated, it leads to a sharpened mind and an enhanced ability to communicate. An over-stimulated Mercury can lead to neurotic behavior, restlessness, and a slightly chaotic mind.

Mercury is weakened in Taurus and Cancer, and somewhat alienated in Scorpio. It is particularly strong – and demanding – in Gemini, also in Virgo, Libra, and to some extent in Aquarius and Pisces.

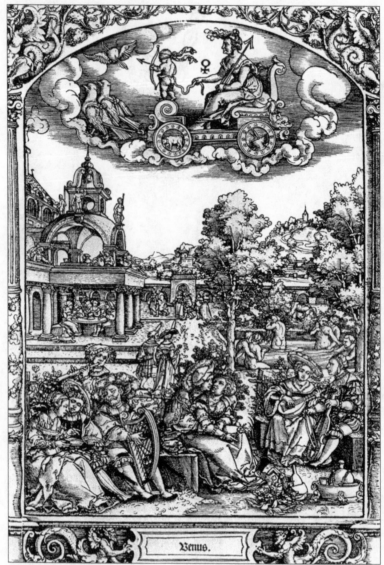

Venus and what it stands for in astrology. Woodcut by Hans Sebald Beham from the 1530's.

Your Health in Your Horoscope

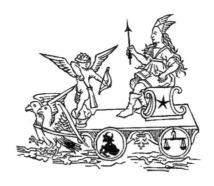

Venus

Venus creates vulnerability and all kinds of minor complications when obstructed. It gives a sense of discomfort, especially in the body part governed by the Zodiac sign it occupies in the horoscope. When enhanced and stimulated, Venus leads to pleasure and well-being, again especially in the body part of its Zodiac sign.

Venus is not that prone to cause trouble, so it needs to be seriously obstructed before it leads to illness or unpleasantness. An over-stimulated Venus can lead to indulgence and one or other kind of gluttony. Loss of self-discipline is also likely.

Venus is not really weakened in any Zodiac sign, except to a minor degree in Aquarius, maybe also a bit unfit for Aries. It is particularly strong – and demanding – in Taurus, Libra, Cancer, and Virgo, but not really to the extent that it gets troublesome.

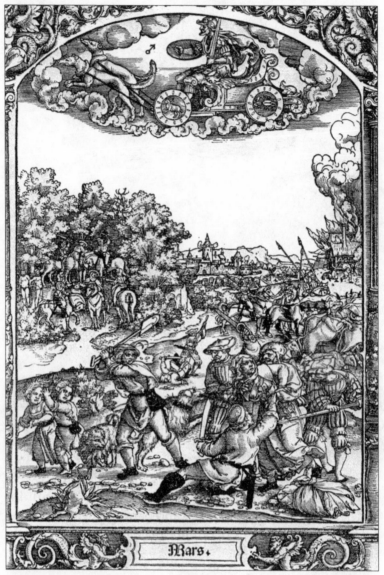

Mars and what it stands for in astrology. Woodcut by Hans Sebald Beham from the 1530's.

Your Health in Your Horoscope

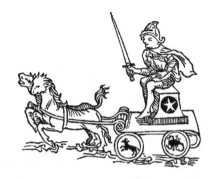

Mars

Mars creates irritation, aggression and pain, when obstructed or held back. It can also cause accidents and dramatic illnesses, although rarely very dangerous ones. They will be somehow connected to the body part governed by the Zodiac sign Mars occupies.

It is important not to block the Mars power too much, or the complications will be severe. Always pay attention to the body part of the Zodiac sign of Mars, and try to find a way of expressing your Mars power better as soon as you sense some trouble with that body part.

An enhanced and stimulated Mars leads to strength, power, and a health that seems to persist just about any threat. An over-stimulated Mars can lead to some manic behavior, loss of temper, even very aggressive impulses. You may become destructive to yourself as well as to others, and there's a risk of wearing yourself down. Mars is just as dangerous when over-stimulated as it is when held back.

Mars is particularly weakened and frustrated in Pisces, to a lesser extent also in Aquarius, Cancer, Taurus and Gemini. It is particularly strong – and demanding – in Aries, Capricorn, Leo, and Sagittarius. Whether weakened or strong, Mars can cause trouble.

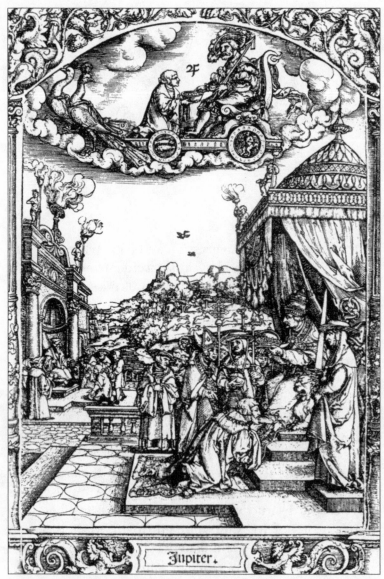

Jupiter and what it stands for in astrology. Woodcut by Hans Sebald Beham from the 1530's.

Your Health in Your Horoscope

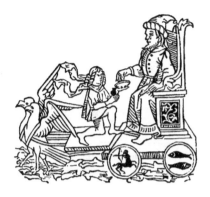

4

Jupiter

Jupiter creates all kinds of complications when held back or seriously obstructed. Things that should be easy become difficult, abilities you can normally trust suddenly fail you, and so on. It's the planet of solutions out of nowhere, so it isn't easily obstructed to the extent that it starts to make trouble. But it can happen – especially if you refuse the successes that seem to befall you out of the blue.

It can also lead to a lack of control of the body part governed by the Zodiac sign the planet occupies.

When enhanced, Jupiter can cure almost any problem or illness, just like that – especially those connected to the body part of its Zodiac sign. An enhanced Jupiter simply makes fate serve you well. An over-stimulated Jupiter can lead to dizziness, inability to focus, and a serious lack of control – especially of the body part governed by the Zodiac sign the planet is in.

Jupiter is slightly weakened in Libra, to some extent also in Aquarius. But the planet is not that out of place in any Zodiac sign. It is particularly strong – and demanding – in Sagittarius, also in Gemini.

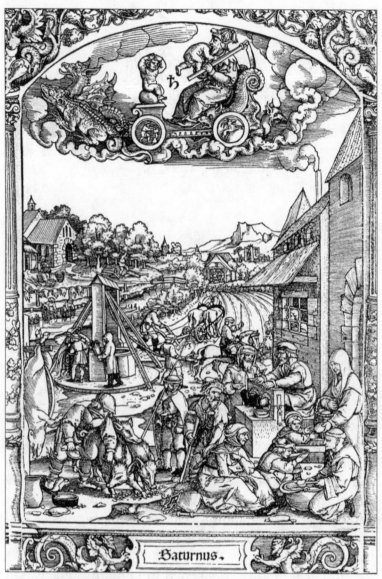

Saturn and what it stands for in astrology. Woodcut by Hans Sebald Beham from the 1530's.

Your Health in Your Horoscope

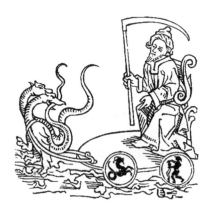

Saturn

Saturn, when obstructed, creates depression and aches that can last very long and go very deep. Saturn can cause very serious and lasting problems, so it should be watched with caution. Mostly, the problems strike at the body part of the Zodiac sign the planet occupies – but not only that. Saturn's malice is capable of reaching beyond single body parts, to affect your life as a whole.

Saturn is still tricky when enhanced and stimulated. It can have side-effects, so to speak. Its power is rather grim by nature. When over-stimulated it can create almost a prison of sorts, a life limited and narrowed down, with burdens or obligations that become too much to carry on your shoulders. This will probably at first be felt as a gnawing discomfort in the body part of its Zodiac sign. Balance your life, so that Saturn doesn't get too much of it.

Saturn is weakened and frustrated in Pisces, Gemini, and Scorpio. It is particularly strong – and demanding – in Capricorn, and to some extent in Aquarius, Libra, and maybe Aries. Whatever Zodiac sign Saturn is in, it can cause serious problems.

Uranus

Uranus creates melancholia and a sense of meaninglessness when obstructed or held back. It can also lead to diminished intellectual capacity and some loss of memory. When stimulated, it causes a contemplative mind, and a gracious attitude toward life. It is a thing of the mind, almost exclusively, whatever body part is governed by its Zodiac sign.

When Uranus is over-stimulated, it can cause confusion, introspection, and a loss of sense of reality, sort of like the mind wandering off in deep meditation. But that's only after quite a lot of over-stimulation, and not necessarily a bad thing.

Uranus is slightly weakened in Taurus and Aries, but not to the extent that it necessarily leads to trouble. It is particularly strong – and demanding – in Aquarius and Sagittarius, also somewhat in Gemini and Libra.

Uranus moves slowly through the Zodiac, taking about seven years to pass a sign. So, its position in the Zodiac is shared by all people born within a few years of each other. Therefore, there are slowly shifting trends in human mentality, also to some extent in ailments of the mind.

Uranus was not discovered until 1781, so there are no older ideas or illustrations of the planet.

Neptune

Neptune creates nightmares and haunting fantasies when obstructed or significantly held back. The ailments and problems it can create are all in the imagination – not just hypochondria, but real mental issues and disorders.

When Neptune is stimulated, it creates splendid dreams, fascinating fantasies, and a rich inner life, with which to enjoy the world even when other things might be demanding. Creativity and its catharsis are also enhanced. Inspiration flows. It's the only planet to bloom in the 12th House.

When over-stimulated, Neptune causes far too vivid dreams and fantasies, risking to tear down the wall between the real and the unreal, so that you might lose contact with reality and the ability to relate to it in a meaningful way.

Neptune is weakened in Taurus, Virgo, and Capricorn, to some extent also in Aries and Libra. It is particularly strong – and demanding – in Pisces and Scorpio, to some extent also in Cancer, Aquarius, and Sagittarius. Neptune can cause real ailments and problems, but only indirectly in other body parts than the brain.

Neptune moves very slowly through the Zodiac, taking almost 14 years to pass through a sign. So, its position in the Zodiac is shared by all people born within several years of each other. Therefore, there are tendencies over time in human dreams, imagination, and artistic preferences. There are similar trends in mental disorders and diseases of the mind, especially disorders that might only be figments of the imagination.

Neptune was not discovered until 1846, so there are no older ideas or illustrations of the planet.

Pluto

Pluto can cause serious accidents and crucial illnesses when severely obstructed or held back. It's a dramatic planet, so it should be handled with care. The changes that Pluto causes tend to be lasting, so ailments of its making might be chronic.

When Pluto is stimulated it can create solutions to problems that seemed impossible, also in the case of illnesses or other health issues. Or it changes other circumstances, so that the problems are no longer of any hindrance.

If over-stimulated, Pluto can cause a chaotic situation where nothing is sure, and nothing seems to be what it should be. That can be quite catastrophic, too, as well as adventurous.

Pluto is weakened and frustrated in Taurus, Virgo, Gemini, and Aquarius. It is particularly strong – and demanding – in Scorpio and Leo, also somewhat in Libra, Aries, and Sagittarius. Whatever Zodiac sign it occupies, Pluto can cause severe and lasting problems.

Pluto is the slowest of the planets, taking 248 years to go through the whole Zodiac. Its elliptic orbit makes the speed vary between 11 and 32 years to pass a sign. So, its position in the Zodiac is shared by all people born within several years of each other. Therefore, there are tendencies in the nature of personal human drama and drastic change, also in diseases – especially the global and most serious ones. The threats to mankind follow the orbit of Pluto.

Pluto was not discovered until 1930, so there are no older ideas or illustrations of the planet.

Your Health in Your Horoscope

AC

Ascendant

The Ascendant (AC) makes you neglect your looks and appearance, when it is obstructed or held back too much. Others will find you less attractive and less sympathetic. When stimulated, it makes you charming and inviting to others. Someone they enjoy to meet, and remember even after a short encounter.

If over-stimulated, the Ascendant can make people take you less seriously, almost like a clown or a caricature.

The Ascendant doesn't cause illnesses or other health problems, but it can make you look like you have them.

The Ascendant is slightly weakened in Pisces and Scorpio, but not significantly so. It is certainly enhanced – and more demanding – in Leo and Aries, also somewhat in Libra and Capricorn. Still, the Ascendant adapts quite well to any Zodiac sign.

MC

Medium Coeli

Medium Coeli (MC) makes you doubt your own capacity and ability, when it is obstructed or held back. You might create problems for yourself just because of your own misunderstandings or pessimistic expectations. You may even develop hypochondria.

If stimulated, MC makes you self-confident and optimistic about your possibilities and abilities. That alone can be enough to grant you success in your efforts. If overstimulated, MC makes you over-confident and unnecessarily daring. You make mistakes by underestimating complications and trusting your abilities almost blindly.

MC doesn't create illnesses by itself, but it can certainly make you believe that you have them.

Medium Coeli is slightly weakened in Scorpio, maybe also in Pisces and Gemini, but not to the extent that it causes problems on its own. It is slightly enhanced in Aquarius and Cancer. But MC really adapts similarly well to any Zodiac sign.

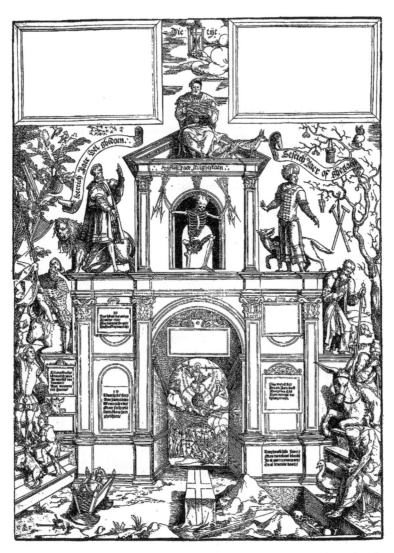

The ages of man, from the cradle to the grave. Illustration by Cornelis Anthonisz, c.1550. In astrology, the ages of man are represented by the planets, traditionally given seven years each in the following order: the moon, Mercury, Venus, the sun, Mars, Jupiter, Saturn, Uranus, Neptune, and Pluto.

Introduction to Medical Astrology   109

The Houses and your health

The Houses of the horoscope show *where* things happen in your life. That's true also for indications about your health.

The twelve Houses are different settings or environments of your life. They are related to the twelve Zodiac signs, but they still function independently. Here are the twelve Houses and keywords to the life environment each of them governs:

House	Keyword
1st House	*Identity*. How others see you.
2nd House	*Resources*. Your personal ability and economy.
3rd House	*Communication*. Your friends and acquaintances, also education.
4th House	*Home*. Your home and family.
5th House	*Pastime*. Your personal preferences, pleasures and interests.
6th House	*Work*. Your profession and daily work.
7th House	*Partners*. Your partners in love and other relations.
8th House	*Unknown*. What you cannot control – fate as well as bloodline.
9th House	*Travel*. Changes of your perspective.
10th House	*Career*. Your social status.
11th House	*Ideals*. Your ideals, and your interaction in the community.
12th House	*Shortcomings*. Your sacrifices, what you are unable to express.

Regarding your health, some of the Houses are far more important than others, but planets in any House can cause illness or other health issues according to the planet and the Zodiac sign it occupies. Such health problems tend to be most evident or cause the most trouble in the life environment of the House in question.

The exceptions are the 12th, 6th, and 8th House, in that order of importance. They reveal something about your general health, whether there are planets inside them or not. Health issues of those Houses rarely get serious without any planet in them, but they still affect your general well-being, although in less dramatic ways.

The 12th House

The 12th House is sometimes dramatically called the Hell of the horoscope. It shows your weakness, what you have to yield in life in order for the rest of your talents to bloom. Therefore, this House shows what parts of your health might be less dependable and more at risk.

To figure that out in your own horoscope, just consider the Zodiac sign occupying the House, and any planets that might be there. The Zodiac sign shows what body part is prone to cause health problems:

Sign	Health issue
Aries	head, brain
Taurus	neck, throat, ears, nose, teeth, hearing
Gemini	lungs, speech, smell
Cancer	skin
Leo	heart, blood
Virgo	food intake intestines
Libra	food processing intestines, excrement
Scorpio	genitals, hormones
Sagittarius	eyes

Capricorn	bones, spine
Aquarius	arms, legs
Pisces	nerves

Any planet in the House shows the type of problems you may get in that body part, especially if the planet is obstructed. Read the previous chapter about the planets and your health to learn more about it. Here are keywords for each planet's possible effect in the 12th House:

Planet	Ailment
Sun	fatigue
Moon	worry
Mercury	uncertainty
Venus	unpleasantness
Mars	accidents
Jupiter	misfortune
Saturn	complications
Uranus	confusion
Neptune	hypochondria
Pluto	malfunction

The Ascendant (AC) is never anything but the cusp of the 1st House, so it is excluded here. Medium Coeli (MC) almost never gets that near the horizon, except maybe on latitudes near the North or South Pole. If it's in the 12th House, it can cause serious loss of trust in your own health or your ability to heal – whether that's true or not. It may even cause you to lose your will to heal.

Remember that the 12th House shows constant weaknesses, which remain all your life. They can sometimes change for the better or the worse, but probably not disappear completely. You do wisely to be aware of them, so as not to challenge your weaknesses too much.

Understanding them will also make it easier for you to come to terms with the conditions you have to accept in your life.

The 6th House

The 6th House is traditionally called the *House of Health*, because of its vast importance to your general well-being. It is actually the House of your work, describing what you do for a living, and how you handle it. Of course, the everyday struggle in your profession is the most important influence on your physical and mental state.

Most work wears us down after decades of daily struggle – some more than others, and in very different ways. If you have a job demanding hard physical activity, it's bound to cause corresponding physical problems at length. Similarly, a job with daily mental strain is sure to take its toll on your psyche.

Contrary to the 12th House, the Zodiac sign in this House indicates a body part of yours that is particularly resourceful and trustworthy, so it will normally take long to give you trouble – but at length it will. So, pay attention to this risk early on, and you can save yourself some serious trouble.

Here are the body parts that are particularly strong, but also strained, in the 6th House:

Sign	Body part
Aries	head, brain
Taurus	neck, throat, ears, nose, teeth, hearing
Gemini	lungs, speech, smell
Cancer	skin
Leo	heart, blood
Virgo	food intake intestines
Libra	food processing intestines, excrement

Scorpio	genitals, hormones
Sagittarius	eyes
Capricorn	bones, spine
Aquarius	arms, legs
Pisces	nerves

Any planet in the 6th House shows increased activity and intensity in your work, whatever it is you do. That means you run a higher risk of tearing down the strength you initially have in the body part of the Zodiac sign the planet occupies. But the planet also specifies what type of problem you can expect when your work is not going as well as it should, or when you allow yourself to get carried away by it.

A planet in the 6th House does not necessarily lead to an illness or other health issue, but it increases the risk – simply because the planet increases the activity of that House. You can read above about the planets and your health to learn more about how the planets function, but here are keywords for each planet and its possible (though not necessary) negative effect on your health in the 6th House:

Planet	Ailment
Sun	exertion
Moon	depression
Mercury	stress
Venus	unpleasantness, nausea
Mars	irritation, pain, accident
Jupiter	exaggeration, loss of control
Saturn	burden, breakdown
Uranus	confusion
Neptune	distraction, alienation
Pluto	destruction

Your Health in Your Horoscope

Neither the Ascendant nor Medium Coeli can ever be in the 6th House, so they are excluded here.

Remember that the 6th House ingredients are normally ones of strength and capacity, and not the opposite. But when going too far, or too long, they can become exhausted and thereby cause serious health issues.

The 8th House

The 8th House is traditionally called the *House of Death*, which is certainly something related to health in many ways. The House indicates, among other things, how you will die.

I know that this is quite serious, so I hesitated about including it. Please don't be alarmed. The House is mainly about things in life that you cannot control at all. The occult and supernatural are here. So are your relatives, because you can't choose them, and death in a symbolic way, since that's also something mostly out of our control – otherwise most of us would keep it off forever.

Since this is the House beyond control, not much can be done about what it shows. But for health considerations, you may want to take extra care of the body function indicated by the Zodiac sign of the 8th House. This may increase your chances of not being struck by that kind of death prematurely. But again: don't let this perspective get to you.

Here are the body types connected to a person's death suggested by the Zodiac sign in the 8th House of that person's horoscope, and more generally speaking the circumstances where death occurs.

Sign	Fatality	Circumstance
Aries	head, brain	activity
Taurus	neck, throat	resting
Gemini	lungs	relaxing

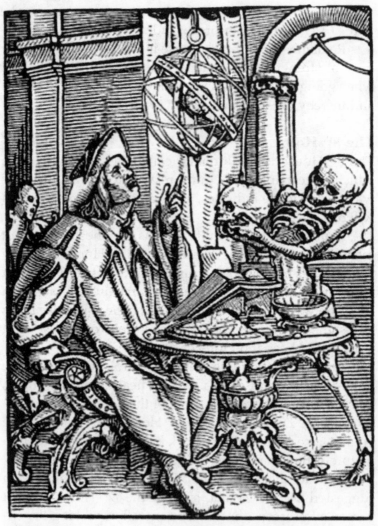

The astrologer and Death. From The Dance of Death by Hans Holbein the Younger, 1538. The joke is that the astrologer is unable to predict his own death.

Cancer	skin	caring
Leo	heart, blood	appearing
Virgo	food intake intestines	working
Libra	food processing intestines	preparing
Scorpio	genitals, hormones	surprise
Sagittarius	eyesight	traveling
Capricorn	bones, spine	struggling
Aquarius	arms, legs, movement	pondering
Pisces	nerves	worrying

Most people die of heart failure, but they don't all have Leo in the 8th House. The House must be understood in a more symbolic way, describing other particular circumstances than just what organ failed.

It must always be remembered in astrology that the components of the horoscope are symbols, indicating forces and tendencies that are not concrete by nature – but they do manifest themselves in concrete ways, now and then. Their concrete manifestations, though, can carry the symbolic meanings in very different ways. There is rarely, if ever, just one concrete manifestation possible. To put it in other words: there are more ways than one to skin a cat.

Any planet in the 8th House may have some influence on the type of death you can expect, but it's far from certain. Many of us have no planets in the 8th House, but we will still die someday.

Some planets indicate other things in the 8th House. For example, the sun in that House suggests a lack of contact with the father, maybe by his early demise. The moon suggests the same about the mother. Of course, these are not decisive indicators. It's just one thing they can imply.

Mars in the 8th House suggest a sudden death. Pluto makes it a complete surprise to all. Venus in the 8th House indicates a painless death. So does Mercury and Jupiter, whereas Saturn tends to suggest the opposite. Neptune would hint at death in one's sleep. Uranus in the House gives awareness of death before it arrives.

Generally speaking, when a planet in the 8th House is active at the moment of death, it suggests the following about that passage:

Planet	Demise
Sun	natural, after exertion
Moon	angst
Mercury	carefree
Venus	painless, peaceful
Mars	sudden
Jupiter	gradual, fortunate
Saturn	troublesome
Uranus	awaited
Neptune	unawares
Pluto	surprising

The Ascendant cannot be anywhere but at the cusp of the 1st House, so it's excluded. Medium Coeli can be in the 8th House, although it's far from common. It indicates that the person feels quite aware of death approaching, and how far or near it is – whether that's accurate or not.

Again, these are suggestions only. Death is a mystery that resists scrutiny.

Other Houses

The other Houses have indirect effects on your health. Mainly, they indicate where you catch a disease or get another health problem. For example, if it's in the 7th House, chances are that you got it from your partner, or the other way around. If it's in the 4th House, you got it in your family or home environment, in the 6th House you got it at work, in the 11th House you got it from a stranger, and so on.

The nature of the disease is shown by the Zodiac sign of that House, and any planet therein.

Here is a list of the Houses, and what they suggest about where or from whom you catch a certain disease:

House	Origin of ailment
1st	Personal habits
2nd	Chronic from birth
3rd	Friends
4th	Home and family
5th	Pastime activities
6th	Work
7th	Partner
8th	Unknown, probably genetic
9th	Travel
10th	Work-place or social life
11th	Strangers, the community
12th	Weakness, low resistance

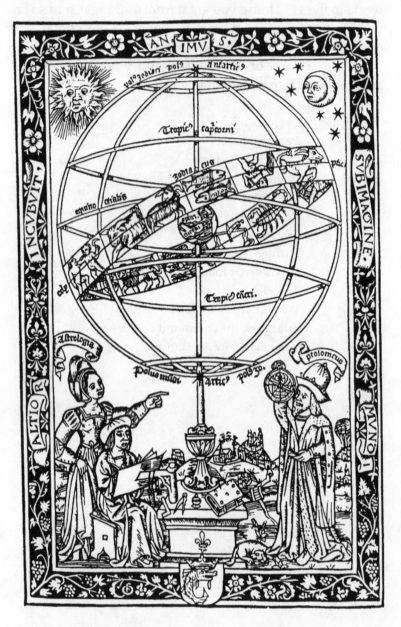

The heavenly spheres. Woodcut by Erhard Schön, 1515.

Your Health in Your Horoscope

The aspects and your health

The planets are the active ingredients in the horoscope, the *what* of any personal talent or event in life. The aspects, special angles that connect them, are the *why*. They explain what dynamics lie behind the characteristics and tendencies of the planets involved.

That *why* works both ways: When two planets are connected with an aspect, each planet's tendencies can be understood by the aspect to the other one. There is no point in trying to decide a first cause between them, since that, too, changes from one situation to another.

In medical astrology, your health is understood much better by studying the aspects. Usually, health problems appear when the two sides of an aspect get unbalanced, so that one side dominates and leaves the other lacking. Two health issues can emerge from this: the weakened side can start to show symptoms, but so can the dominant side – from over-stimulation.

Aspects happen between planets or astrological points. Still, the Zodiac signs and Houses of those planets need to be considered for a better understanding of the consequences. They show the *how* and *where* of the effects.

Here are the major aspects and keywords for the effects they have on planets connected by them:

Aspect	Effect
conjunction, 0°	blending
opposition, 180°	separation
trine, 120°	harmony
square, 90°	conflict
sextile, 60°	cooperation

♂

Conjunction

Conjunction is when two or more planets are very close to one another in the horoscope chart. Astrologically, this means that their powers blend, so that they sort of form a new planet with its own distinct traits.

As for your health, the conjunction creates a point of great power in your horoscope. Normally, it will mean strength, and not weakness, but it is also a very demanding force. Therefore, it can cause serious problems when obstructed or held back. A conjunction needs to be lived out, or it will sort of backfire.

On the other hand, an over-stimulated conjunction can also lead to health issues. This is actually more likely than the conjunction being obstructed or restrained, since it is such a power in the horoscope – easier to overdo than to suppress.

Here are keywords for what the planets might cause when over-stimulated by a conjunction or obstructed by another aspect:

Planet	Over-stimulation	Obstruction
Sun	exertion	fatigue
Moon	desperation	anxiety
Mercury	stress	confusion
Venus	discomfort	dissatisfaction
Mars	strain	pain
Jupiter	exaggeration	misfortune
Saturn	burden	disappointment
Uranus	bewilderment	mistake
Neptune	distraction	boredom
Pluto	destruction	complication
Ascendant	pompousness	unattractiveness
Medium Coeli	self-indulgence	misunderstanding

Some of the above express themselves mentally, but can still show physical symptoms. Those are the moon, Mercury, Uranus, Neptune, AC, and MC. Other planets express themselves mentally or physically according to the Zodiac sign they occupy.

To know the health hazards of a conjunction, it's easy enough to consider the Zodiac sign involved. Usually it's just one – if not two planets are really close, but still in different signs.

Here are keywords for the body parts that the Zodiac signs govern, which may be afflicted by a conjunction of planets that is over-stimulated, or obstructed by another aspect:

Sign	Health issue
Aries	head, brain
Taurus	neck, throat, ears, nose, teeth, hearing
Gemini	lungs, speech, smell
Cancer	skin
Leo	heart, blood
Virgo	food intake intestines
Libra	food processing intestines, excrement
Scorpio	genitals, hormones
Sagittarius	eyes
Capricorn	bones, spine
Aquarius	arms, legs
Pisces	nerves

The House is also plain to see, usually being just one. It shows where the conjunction health problems may emerge, what part of life triggers them. Here is a list of the Houses, and what they suggest about where or from whom you catch a certain disease:

House	Origin of ailment
1st	Personal habits
2nd	Chronic from birth
3rd	Friends
4th	Home and family
5th	Pastime activities
6th	Work
7th	Partner
8th	Unknown, probably genetic
9th	Travel
10th	Work-place or social life
11th	Strangers, the community
12th	Weakness, low resistance

It is significantly more difficult to understand and interpret the power formed by the actual conjunct planets. You have to contemplate the characteristics of each planet involved, and come up with what that leads to in their blending. The possible combinations are too many to go through here. Check the keywords for the planets above.

For example, an obstructed sun can lead to fatigue, and an obstructed moon to anxiety. So, the combined effect might be a depression difficult to snap out of. A serious loss of confidence. When over-stimulated, the same aspect might lead to wearing oneself down both physically and emotionally, maybe even falling into panic. That's cause for a time-out and patient recreation.

Mercury leads to confusion when obstructed, and Saturn to disappointment. Together they suggest a lack of control of one's fate, a certain incompetence. Over-stimulated they may lead to overload and personal crisis. That's what some people experience when they allow themselves to be consumed by their career, until they have a breakdown.

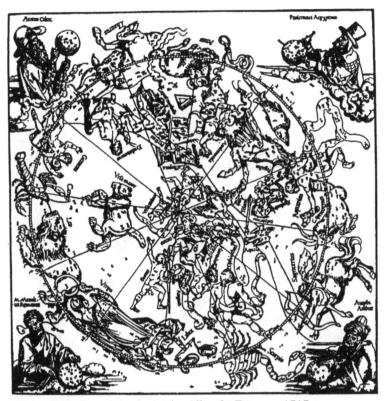

The constellations. Woodprint by Albrecht Dürer c. 1515.

Use your imagination to figure out the significance of the other conjunctions, as you come across them in your own or someone else's horoscope.

Opposition

Opposition is when two planets are on opposite sides of the horoscope chart – approximately 180° apart. The significance of this aspect is pretty much the same as its name: opposition, two interests colliding, so that it's either one or the other, rarely both at work at a given time.

The opposition is almost as powerful in the horoscope as the conjunction, and of great importance for your health. The two sides of the opposition are sort of at war with one another, so when one is dominating, the other suffers and will lead to some health problems. Another time their roles are reversed.

You can probably see in the horoscope what side will usually dominate: the strongest one. For example, if one side of the opposition is a conjunction of two or more planets, it will surely be the dominant one during most of your life. The other side will only take over at short periods, when stimulated by other events or forces.

The same is true for a planet that has several other aspects to other planets in the horoscope. That also increases its power, so it will be the more dominant one. When the powers on both sides of the opposition are rather equal, the dominance will swing back and forth, leading to several complications in your life, and health risks at both sides.

An opposition rarely creates over-stimulation of the involved planets, but easily obstruction to one or both sides of it. So, here are the planets and how they react when obstructed:

Planet	Obstruction
Sun	fatigue
Moon	anxiety
Mercury	confusion

Your Health in Your Horoscope

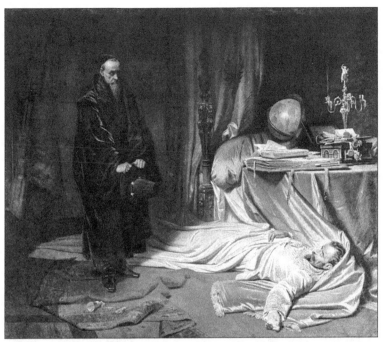

The astrologer Seni watches the dead body of murdered Albrecht von Wallenstein. Painting by Karl von Piloty, 1855.

Venus	dissatisfaction
Mars	pain
Jupiter	misfortune
Saturn	disappointment
Uranus	mistake
Neptune	boredom
Pluto	complication
Ascendant (AC)	unattractiveness
Medium Coeli (MC)	misunderstanding

To understand the health issues, consider the planets involved, the Zodiac signs they are in, and the Houses they occupy. Use the keywords listed above to make your interpretation of the ingredients easier.

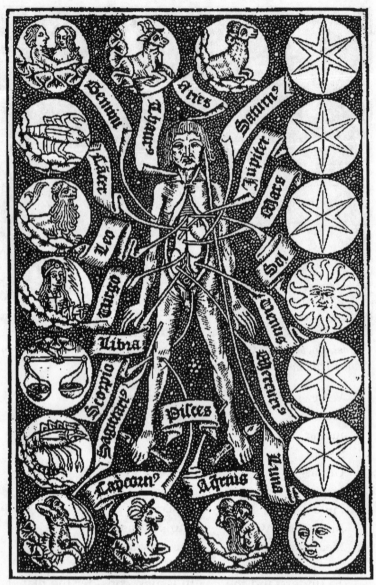

Zodiac Man, with Zodiac signs as well as the planets linked to them marked out. From The Shepherds Calendar, c.1495.

Your Health in Your Horoscope

Trine

Trine is when two planets are about 120° apart. This is an aspect of harmony, so that the two involved sides coexist smoothly. They stimulate one another, although usually not in a very concrete way.

The positive power of this aspect makes it unlikely to cause serious health problems. Instead, it makes the involved planets increasingly beneficial, so that illness is less likely than it would be without them – illness of the Zodiac signs and Houses they occupy, that is. The rest of the horoscope is unaffected.

Of course it can happen at times that one side of the trine dominates to the extent that the other side is obstructed or neglected. Then the latter can cause some ailment, but rarely anything serious. Check the lists with keywords above to figure out what that can lead to, but with trines only to a minor extent.

What is more likely is that they over-stimulate one another, so that both can express such symptoms, according to the characteristics of the involved planets, Zodiac signs, and Houses.

Here are keywords for what the planets might cause when over-stimulated, although with trines it rarely goes to any extremes:

Planet	Over-stimulation
Sun	exertion
Moon	anxiety
Mercury	stress
Venus	discomfort
Mars	strain
Jupiter	exaggeration

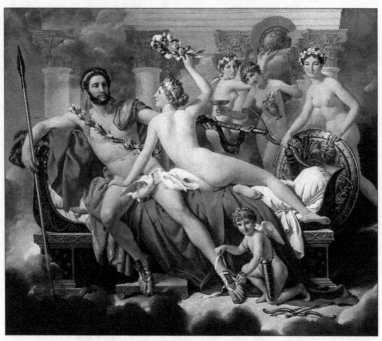

Mars, the god of war, being seduced by Venus, the goddess of love. Painting by Jacques-Louis David, 1824.

Saturn	burden
Uranus	bewilderment
Neptune	distraction
Pluto	deterioration
Ascendant (AC)	pompousness
Medium Coeli (MC)	self-indulgence

An aspect figure that appears now and then is the *Big Trine*, where planets on three locations in the horoscope are connected with trines. That makes a triangle covering the whole horoscope circle. This increases the power and activity of the involved planets considerably, so the risk of over-stimulation also rises. Normally, though, such an aspect figure improves one's health.

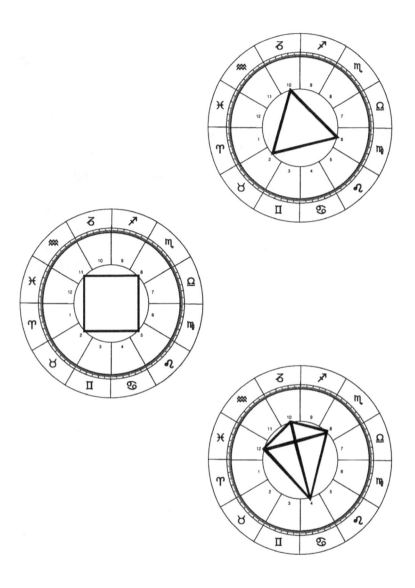

Three aspect figures of the horoscope. From top to bottom: the big trine, the big square (which usually also has two oppositons), and the kite (combining two sextiles, two trines, a square, and an opposition).

Introduction to Medical Astrology 131

Square

Square is the aspect when planets are about 90° apart. This is a complication, where the planets involved are in conflict, working in separate directions or outright against one another. It's a stimulating and constructive aspect, but also one that easily leads to trouble. Much is done by it, but nothing is easy.

The health is at some risk, on both sides of the aspect. Usually both sides experience problems and health issues to about the same extent, but if one side is dominant the other is sure to suffer more. Still, no side is ever completely without problems.

See the keyword lists below for how the planets behave when obstructed by this aspect:

Planet	Obstruction
Sun	fatigue
Moon	frustration
Mercury	confusion
Venus	dissatisfaction
Mars	pain
Jupiter	misfortune
Saturn	disappointment
Uranus	mistake
Neptune	angst
Pluto	complication
Ascendant (AC)	unattractiveness
Medium Coeli (MC)	misunderstanding

It is also possible that a square over-stimulates both sides of it, but that is rare. A square creates conflicts that takes their toll on both sides. There is rarely an opportunity for any of the involved planets to excel.

Your Health in Your Horoscope

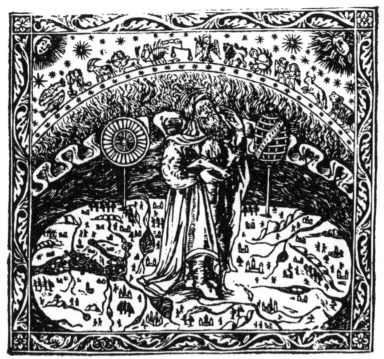

The Greek mathematician Archimedes on a flat Earth, surrounded by the elements and the heavenly spheres. Woodcut from 1503.

In some horoscopes there can be four square aspects connecting planets into a complete geometric figure covering the whole horoscope chart. That's called the *Big Square*, and it's rather rare. In such an aspect figure, all the involved planets are likely to be over-stimulated, at least at times, and your health can be at risk at all the four spots.

Notice also that a Big Square has two oppositions crossing the aspect figure diagonally. These aspects are even more important, and tend to dominate events. If you have a Big Square, there's a great risk that you repeatedly wear yourself out.

Sextile

Sextile is the aspect where planets are about 60° apart. It is a positive aspect, giving a creative boost to both sides of it. They cooperate naturally, inspiring each other to additional feats and heightened activity. It's an aspect through which much gets done – like a charm.

The sextile is not likely to cause any serious health problems, ever. It may occasionally trigger some over-stimulation, but that's rare. It's even more rare that it creates obstacles for one of the involved planets, or holds anything back.

At times there can be some unbalance in a sextile, so that one side gets somewhat dominant, and the other suffers. But that's temporary, and should not lead to any lasting discomfort.

The only exception is if one side of the sextile is enforced by additional planets in a conjunction, or by a number of aspects to other parts of the horoscope. Then the other side of the aspect might get kind of drained, working almost exclusively for the dominant side of the sextile. The losing side will at length cause some health issues. Again, this is not likely to develop into something very serious – but in the long run, it could.

NICOLAI COPERNICI

net, in quo terram cum orbe lunari tanquam epicyclo contineri
diximus. Quinto loco Venus nono menfe reducitur. Sextum
deniç locum Mercurius tenet, octuaginta dierum fpacio circu
currens. In medio uero omnium refidet Sol. Quis enim in hoc

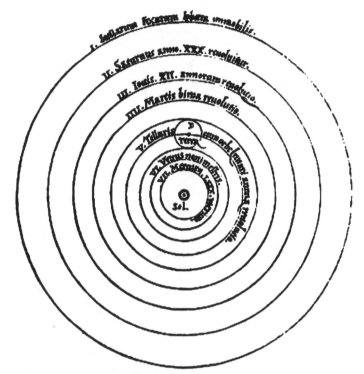

pulcherimo templo lampadem hanc in alio uel meliori loco po
neret, quàm unde totum fimul pofsit illuminare? Siquidem non
inepte quidam lucernam mundi, alŋ mentem, alŋ rectorem uo-
cant. Trimegiftus uifibilem Deum, Sophoclis Electra intuentē
omnia. Ita profecto tanquam in folio regali Sol refidens circum
agentem gubernat Aftrorum familiam. Tellus quoç minime
fraudatur lunari minifterio, fed ut Ariftoteles de animalibus
ait, maximā Luna cū terra cognationē habet. Concipit interea à

Page from De revolutionibus orbium coelestium by Copernicus 1543,
where he argued for a heliocentric solar system.

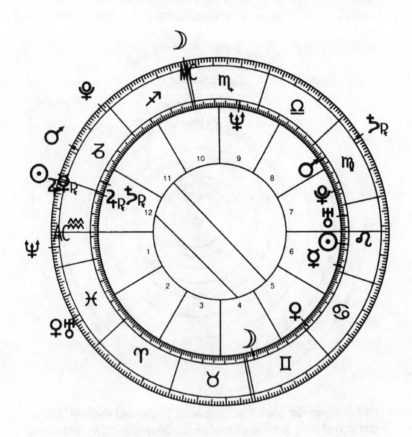

Transit chart for Barack Obama at the time of his inauguration, on January 20, 2009, at 12 noon, because that was the time he took over as President. The transit planets are outside the outer circle, and Obama's native planets inside. The aspects between them are marked by lines in the innermost circle, except for the conjunctions, which are visible anyway. There are several important conjunctions to Obama's horoscope at this moment, but only two other aspects – at the narrow orb allowed here.

Your Health in Your Horoscope

The transits and your health

When planets moving in their orbits in the sky form aspects, special angles, with planets or similar points in the horoscope, these are called *transits*, i.e. transiting or passing aspects.

The aspects within your horoscope chart are fixed, remaining the same all your life, and therefore indicating dynamics that you will experience all through. The transits, though, are passing things. The duration of a transit depends on the speed of the planet involved. That differs tremendously. The moon moves through a transit in a couple of hours, whereas Pluto, the slowest of the planets, takes about a year to do the same.

A quick transit has a passing effect in your life, but the slow ones mark changes that last for long, or even for good.

Here is the approximate time it takes each planet and other astrological point to travel through the whole Zodiac, from a geocentric perspective:

Planet	Orbit
Sun	1 year
Moon	1 month
Mercury	1 year
Venus	1 year
Mars	2 years
Jupiter	12 years
Saturn	29 years
Uranus	84 years
Neptune	164 years
Pluto	248 years

So, the moon goes through every possible transit aspect with your horoscope each month, and the sun each year. But Uranus takes a lifetime to do the same, and with Pluto you will only experience some of its possible transits.

The Ascendant and Medium Coeli can also be seen to move through the Zodiac, but they are not used in transits.

These are the basic aspects to consider when they form transits with planets and astrological points in your horoscope, and keywords for what they generally represent:

Aspect	Effect
conjunction, 0°	blending
opposition, 180°	separation
trine, 120°	harmony
square, 90°	conflict
sextile, 60°	cooperation

For transit aspects, a narrow *orb* is to be used. The orb is the distance from the exact angle allowed for an aspect to count as such. Whatever the kind of aspect, in transits the orb should be no more than 1°. The transit can be felt slightly beforehand, especially if it's a slow planet, but its peak starts when it reaches that close to the planet in your native chart. Of course, its effect may remain very long afterward.

Here is a list of the transiting planets, and keywords to their influence on the planets or astrological points of the horoscope chart that they form aspects with:

Transit	Influence
Sun	concentration
Moon	urge
Mercury	attention
Venus	attraction

Mars	resolution
Jupiter	luck
Saturn	duty
Uranus	contemplation
Neptune	fantasy
Pluto	catharsis

And here's a list of the native chart planets and points, with keywords for health issues that may arise when triggered by some transit aspects:

Native	Ailment
Sun	fatigue
Moon	anxiety
Mercury	uncertainty
Venus	discomfort
Mars	irritation
Jupiter	misfortune
Saturn	complication
Uranus	confusion
Neptune	hypochondria
Pluto	malfunction
Ascendant	self-neglect
Medium Coeli	self-doubt

Here are the Zodiac signs and the body parts they govern, where health issues may appear through some transit aspects to a planet or point therein:

Sign	Health issue
Aries	head, brain
Taurus	neck, throat, ears, nose, teeth, hearing
Gemini	lungs, speech, smell
Cancer	skin

Leo	heart, blood
Virgo	food intake intestines
Libra	food processing intestines, excrement
Scorpio	genitals, hormones
Sagittarius	eyes
Capricorn	bones, spine
Aquarius	arms, legs
Pisces	nerves

The conjunction is by far the most important transit aspect, much more influential than the others. Especially conjunctions formed by the slow planets, Saturn, Uranus, Neptune, and Pluto, mark life-changing events, although not always that easy to recognize at the moment they happen. Often their effects become evident only in distant retrospect.

The opposition is also quite strong and important. The square transit usually expresses itself very concretely, so its effect is easy to observe. The trine and the sextile, though, are not always that evident. Mainly, they create a good mood and help you get things done. You might tend to see these effects as bursts of inspiration, or what is nowadays often called flow.

Regarding your health, the transits can create imbalances in your life and personality, which might in turn trigger health issues. Here are the transit aspects, and how they influence your health:

♂

Conjunction

Conjunction is when the transit planet and a planet or astrological point in your horoscope are at the same position. It's the strongest of the transits, and its effect is often obvious even when the transiting planet is quick in its orbit.

The conjunction transit gives a boost to the planet it passes over. It doesn't obstruct or hold back that power, but there is a clear risk that it will be over-stimulated.

Here is a list of the native chart planets, and what health issues they might cause when over-stimulated in a transit conjunction:

Native	Over-stimulation
Sun	exertion
Moon	desperation
Mercury	stress
Venus	discomfort
Mars	strain
Jupiter	exaggeration
Saturn	burden
Uranus	bewilderment
Neptune	distraction
Pluto	destruction
Ascendant	pompousness
Medium Coeli	self-indulgence

To learn more about possible over-stimulation in a transit conjunction, consider what transiting planet is involved and check the list with keywords for transit planet influences below.

Contrary to conjunctions within your native chart, the transit doesn't cause a blending of the planetary forces involved. The transit planet represents an event that your native chart planet benefits from, without any merging taking place. Things go your way. The transit conjunction can also indicate a success or breakthrough of some kind, without any outer events causing it.

Use the list of keywords below to figure out what kind of influence the transiting planet has in the conjunction:

Transit	Influence
Sun	concentration
Moon	urge
Mercury	attention
Venus	attraction
Mars	resolution
Jupiter	luck
Saturn	duty
Uranus	contemplation
Neptune	fantasy
Pluto	catharsis

As for the effect on your life, study the planet or astrological point in your birth chart that is involved in the transit conjunction, also its Zodiac sign and House.

Opposition

Opposition is when the transit planet and a planet or astrological point in your horoscope are about 180° apart, opposite one another. It's the second strongest transit aspect, and usually quite distinct in its effect, also when it comes to health issues.

The transiting planet shows that something happens in the House it passes through, which becomes an obstacle to what the opposed planet in the horoscope chart is about. By checking the Houses involved in particular, it can often be quite evident what will happen, at least in a general sense.

Each of the twelve Houses in the horoscope is in natural opposition to the House on the other side of it, so that the 1st House opposes the 7th House, and so on.

When you consider what life-environment each House signifies, these oppositions are easy to understand. For example, the 1st House deals with the personality of the individual, which is naturally opposed to the 7th House showing partnership commitments. In any partnership, you need to sacrifice some personal interests. If you don't, the partnership will surely suffer.

Here are the twelve Houses and keywords for the life-environment each one represents, ordered so that the opposing ones are on the same line:

House	Keyword	House	Keyword
1st	Identity	7th	Partners
2nd	Resources	8th	Unknown
3rd	Communication	9th	Travel
4th	Home	10th	Career
5th	Pastime	11th	Ideals
6th	Work	12th	Shortcomings

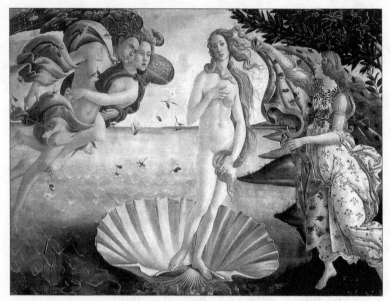

The birth of the goddess Venus, by Sandro Botticelli c. 1485.

Some health problems are likely to appear, especially if the transiting planet is a slow and strong one. The transiting moon does little more than accomplish momentary mood-swings, but all the planets from Mars to Pluto have a more distinct and lasting effect on your health. The slower the planet, the longer the effect lasts.

The body part governed by the Zodiac sign that the transiting planet occupies is rarely affected at all. It's the opposite planet, the one in your horoscope chart, which is obstructed, and therefore also the one causing health problems. Consider what planet it is, and what sign and House it occupies, to learn more about the health problem that might appear.

Your Health in Your Horoscope

Trine

Trine is when the transit planet and a planet or astrological point in your horoscope are about 120° apart. It's the third aspect in strength, but its effects are quite vague and difficult to ascertain. It creates harmony between its two sides, inspiring them to increased achievements. It shows that there is no conflict between them.

Therefore, it's not likely that the trine causes any kind of problem. Instead, it's an aspect stimulating solutions.

The astrological Houses of the horoscope have natural trine relations: The 1st House is in trine with the 5th House and the 9th House, the 2nd House is in trine with the 6th and the 10th, and so on.

When you compare the life-environments of the Houses in trine, you can see their positive relations.

For example, your personal identity (1st House) is what you get to express in your pastime (5th House), and your travel and other changes you allow yourself (9th House) will increase your ability to present yourself to others – not to mention that they add excitement to your pastime.

Below are the twelve Houses and their keywords, arranged so that the ones in trine are on the same line. Observe that all three Houses on a line are in trine to one another:

H.	Keyword	H.	Keyword	H.	Keyword
1st	Identity	5th	Pastime	9th	Travel
2nd	Resources	6th	Work	10th	Career
3rd	Communication	7th	Partners	11th	Ideals
4th	Home	8th	Unknown	12th	Shortcomings

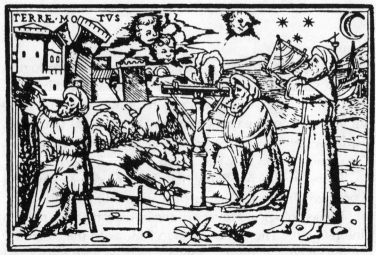

Arabian astrologers examining the sky. Illustration from In somnium scipionis by Ambrosius Macrobius, in an edition from 1513.

It's very unlikely that a transit trine would create obstacles for the planet in the horoscope chart. So, in that way a trine would not cause health problems. What could happen is that the native planet gets over-stimulated, in which case you should examine that planet, and the Zodiac sign and House it occupies, to figure out the effect.

But a trine over-stimulation, too, is not likely to cause any serious or lasting health problems. Probably no more than some discomfort while the transit lasts.

Your Health in Your Horoscope

◻

Square

Square is when the transit planet and a planet or point in your horoscope are about 90° apart. The square tends to lead to concrete effects that are hard to ignore. It's not necessarily for the bad, although that can certainly happen, but it leads to sudden events and some intensified activity.

Something happens that forces you to respond. It might also sabotage things you have going for you. The square is an event happening in one field of your life, the consequences of which are felt in some other part of your life.

Of course, the nature of the event can be learned from the transiting planet and the Zodiac sign and House it occupies at the time of the transit. The major effect it has on your life is seen on the planet in your native chart that the transit forms its square with. It can be further understood by considering the Zodiac sign and House occupied by your native planet.

Notice that the twelve Houses of the horoscope have natural squares, i.e. conflicting interests that are both stimulating and troublesome. Here are the Houses, keywords for their environments, and their squares:

House	Keyword	Square Houses
1st	Identity	4th and 10th
2nd	Resources	5th and 11th
3rd	Communication	6th and 12th
4th	Home	7th and 1st
5th	Pastime	8th and 2nd
6th	Work	9th and 3rd
7th	Partners	10th and 4th
8th	Unknown	11th and 5th
9th	Travel	12th and 6th

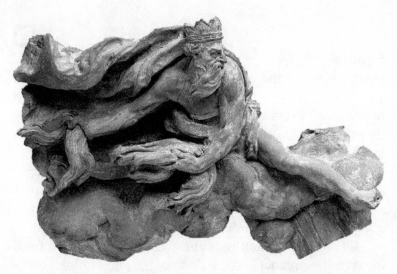

The god Jupiter casting a thunderbolt. Relief by Luc Faydherbe, c. 1650.

10th	Career	1st and 7th
11th	Ideals	2nd and 8th
12th	Shortcomings	3rd and 9th

So, your personal identity (1st House) is at conflict with your family life (4th House), which tends to demand adaption, and to your social career (10th House) that restrains your behavior. Your personal resources (2nd House) are in conflict with your spare time activities (5th House), which can become costly, and your ideals (11th House), because they demand some sacrifice of you. And so on.

Transit squares do tend to cause some health issues, and when they do it's almost always in the area described by the native planet they form the aspect with. The reverse, health issues on the side of the transiting planet, would only happen when other aspects indicate it, or when the native planet is so strong that it doesn't yield to the square at all.

Sextile

Sextile is when the transit planet and a planet or astrological point in your horoscope are about 60° apart. This is an aspect of creativity and inspirational impulses. It makes things work smoothly and lead effortlessly to fortunate results.

So, regarding health the sextile is much more likely to increase it than cause any problems to it. Not only is the sextile unlikely to cause illnesses and such, it is also too weak to initiate any serious problems. Therefore, the sextile is just as unlikely to cause over-stimulation.

In a transit sextile, the transiting planet represents something happening, which facilitates or solves expressions of the aspected planet in your native chart. The only health problem this can bring is maybe some exertion on the side of the native planet. If so, it's still mild and passes quickly. Check the native planet, its Zodiac sign and House, to learn more about how you might exert yourself.

Since the sextile is more of an asset than a burden, it is more likely to bring on cures to health problems. So, if you had a health issue expressed by the native chart planet, it may get eased or cured by what the transit sextile introduces.

Here are the planets, and the health problems they might cause, which could be eased or solved by a transit sextile to them:

Native	Ailment
Sun	fatigue
Moon	anxiety
Mercury	uncertainty
Venus	discomfort

Mars	pain
Jupiter	misfortune
Saturn	complication
Uranus	confusion
Neptune	angst
Pluto	malfunction
Ascendant	self-neglect
Medium Coeli	self-doubt

And here are the Zodiac signs and the body parts they govern, where health issues may be eased or solved by a transit sextile:

Sign	Health issue
Aries	head, brain
Taurus	neck, throat, ears, nose, teeth, hearing
Gemini	lungs, speech, smell
Cancer	skin
Leo	heart, blood
Virgo	food intake intestines
Libra	food processing intestines, excrement
Scorpio	genitals, hormones
Sagittarius	eyes
Capricorn	bones, spine
Aquarius	arms, legs
Pisces	nerves

So, when a strong sextile appears to a problem spot in your horoscope, be open to solutions that may present themselves in the process.

Diseases in your horoscope

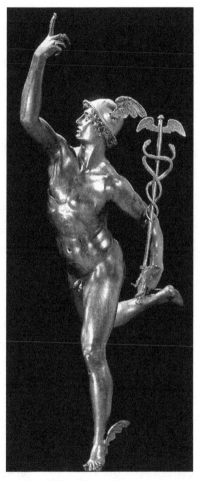

Mercury (Hermes), the god of medicine. He holds the caduce, a winged staff with two serpents twined around it. According to the myth, he stopped two fighting snakes by throwing the staff between them. It has become a sybol of medicine. Statue by Giovanni da Bologna, 1580.

Diseases in your horoscope

Most diseases have particular traits that connect them to certain planets, Zodiac signs, and Houses of the horoscope. Still, astrology is complex. The horoscope has many different ways to describe what seems to be exactly the same – simply because it isn't. One disease can have different symptoms, and be experienced very differently by people who get it.

So, the following are suggestions only, regarding a few well-known diseases and health problems. Life in all its variety doesn't allow for any trustworthy rationalization. See what I say below as suggestions only, examples to give you a better understanding of astrology at work. And please, trust your doctor more than your horoscope!

Common cold

The common cold is rarely serious enough to last more than a week or so, and it is usually not remembered any longer. So, it doesn't involve anyone of the slow outer planets. Also, we tend to get it frequently, maybe annually or more. Again, this suggests the faster planets inside Earth's orbit.

Both Venus and Mercury follow the sun's annual pattern. Venus is beneficial by nature, so it brings problems only when over-stimulated in the birth chart. A transit Venus in itself brings only good things. The sun, though, can bring both strengths and weaknesses, depending on its aspect to a native planet. So can Mercury.

Mercury is particularly relevant to the common cold,

since it is quick and light, but still sometimes distracting, maybe even annoying. Like a cold.

So, both the sun and Mercury, especially the latter, can cause a cold. This might happen when they transit with a square or opposition to a relevant point in the native chart – such as the sun, which controls one's stamina, or Mercury, because of its own character, or the sign Taurus, governing the throat and the nose, or Gemini, governing breathing and smell.

For example, a period when we're all sensitive to the cold is when the sun passes through Scorpio and Sagittarius, which are in opposition to Taurus and Gemini. That's in the fall, from October 23 to December 21. It's a typical time for colds and flus of some distinction.

Quickly passing colds are common when the sun forms a square to Taurus or Gemini – i.e. when it is in Leo and Virgo, also Aquarius and Pisces. That's July 23 to September 22, and January 20 to March 20.

If you have your native sun or Mercury in Taurus or Gemini, you're particularly likely to catch a cold in those periods. In that case you can also catch a particularly annoying cold when transit Mars forms a square or opposition to your sun or Mercury.

If your 12th House is in Taurus or Gemini, you're quite sensitive to the cold and the flu – even if neither Mercury nor the sun is there. That's also the case, although to a lesser extent, if you have your 6th House in Taurus or Gemini.

If none of the above is true for you, and you have no other complications in Taurus or Gemini – such as Mars, Saturn, or a planet with troublesome aspects to it – you probably almost never catch a cold, even when just about everyone around you does.

Cancer
There is no relation between the disease Cancer and the Zodiac sign with the same name. That's just coincidence. The sign Cancer governs the skin, so the only cancer it would be directly linked to is skin cancer.

The nature of cancer is one of uncontrolled growth of cells. Such a process is connected to Jupiter, the planet of expansion. But cancer is also painful, very disturbing and detrimental, mostly lethal, which connects it to Saturn and Pluto. Mars is not enough, although it can trigger changes in the evolvement of the disease.

A cancer that commenced with a Mars transit is likely to be cured, maybe even quite quickly, but one starting with a Saturn transit is more serious and difficult, and one commencing with a Pluto transit is likely to be fatal, at least of lifelong influence.

Since cancer can hit almost any body part, it is not linked to any particular Zodiac sign. But of course, cancer that strikes a certain body part should be noticeable in the Zodiac sign of that organ:

Sign	Health issue
Aries	head, brain
Taurus	neck, throat, ears, nose
Gemini	lungs
Cancer	skin
Leo	blood
Virgo	food intake intestines
Libra	food processing intestines
Scorpio	genitals
Sagittarius	eyes
Capricorn	bones, spine
Aquarius	arms, legs
Pisces	nerves

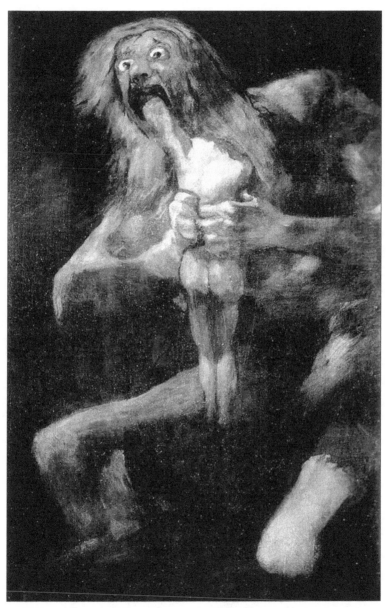

*The god Saturn devouring his son. Wall painting by Francisco Goya,
somewhere between 1819-1823, in his late years.*

Of course, some of the organs above are never struck by cancer.

Some kinds of cancer are more common than others. That differs between the sexes, and has a lot to do with cultural ingredients, pollution, and so on. The slow outer planets signal tendencies in society as a whole, so especially Pluto should be observed for mortality tendencies. That does not necessarily mean cancer, but some cancer forms would be more likely with Pluto in the signs governing the organs they strike.

When Pluto travels through a Zodiac sign, diseases connected to its body part are likely to emerge. But they can also strike persons born in that period, any time during their lives.

For example, when Pluto was in Gemini, 1884-1914, lung cancer would have risen. It also followed the generation born at that time, like some kind of plague. Pluto was in Cancer from 1914, when World War I started (and mustard gas plagued the soldiers). That brought serious skin diseases. Breast cancer, too, is most likely to have emerged in this period. In 1939, when World War II started, Pluto entered Leo, the sign governing the heart and blood, triggering fatal diseases of those kinds, for example leukemia. Stomach cancer might have risen with Pluto in Virgo, 1957-1972, and prostate cancer with Libra in 1972-1984.

Pluto was in Scorpio 1984-1995, which caused no cancer that we know of yet, if not prostate cancer belongs to this sign rather than to Libra. But AIDS emerged in this period, and that's certainly a Scorpio thing.

In 1995 Pluto entered Sagittarius, which could lead to serious eye and eyesight diseases. I thought that solar radiation and the weakened ozone layer would strike, but that seems not to have happened yet. We still have to see what diseases the generation born in that period will be tormented by.

In 2008 Pluto entered Capricorn, which governs the bones and the spine. We have yet to see what that will lead to.

But everyone doesn't get the Pluto disease of the time. Other things in the horoscope must enhance its destructive ability, for example malicious aspects with other forceful planets, like Saturn, Jupiter, and Mars. The sun, too, is an additional indicator if in square or opposition to Pluto in the native chart.

Also the 8th House should be studied, since cancer is frequently a fatal disease, and that's one topic of this House.

Something as varied as cancer is hard to pin down in the horoscope, because it strikes so differently. That means it can show up very differently in people's charts.

Maybe the best clue is the role of Jupiter, the planet of expansion. If it is seriously afflicted by malicious aspects from, say, Pluto or Saturn, maybe Mars too, then the risk of cancer in the organ governed by the Zodiac sign Jupiter occupies should be considered – especially if Jupiter is in the 8th, 12th, or 6th House. But if there's no special cancer that can strike the organ of that Zodiac sign, then the risk for one is minimal.

Bone fracture

Breaking a leg or an arm is a violent misfortune, happening in an instant – so Mars is likely to be involved, probably transit Mars forming a square aspect to your native sun or another planet in your horoscope of some significance. That depends on how the accident affects your life.

If your convalescence obstructs an important activity or plan of yours, the Mars transit is probably pointing to the place in your horoscope representing that activity. It may also point to the 6th House, since the fracture surely impairs your efforts at work. The Mars transit will point to the House governing the life-environment that is the most troubled by the accident.

Capricorn is the Zodiac sign governing the bones of your body, so it should somehow be involved in most cases – either as the sign transit Mars is in, or the sign of the planet that transit Mars aspects.

I say Mars repeatedly, but other planets in transit can cause the same – mainly Saturn and Pluto. In those cases the fracture is sure to be severe and take time to heal.

If the actual moment of the fracture is not a very dramatic experience, then completely different planets and Zodiac signs may be involved – those describing your actual experience of the whole thing more relevantly. For example, if the fracture was not that painful or traumatic, but the most disturbing consequence of it was the loss of a career opportunity for you, then the 10th House of your native chart would be involved. If it ruined a love affair you had going, the 7th House could be involved, also Venus.

The important thing to consider is how the fracture actually affects your life.

Allergy

There are lots of different allergies, but what most of them have in common is an overreaction to a substance or phenomenon, resulting in a certain bodily discomfort.

As for what body part is affected, check the Zodiac sign that governs it. For example, a rash or another skin reaction would be Cancer, whereas nose and throat problems belong to Taurus. Not all body parts are sensitive to allergies, so several Zodiac signs are not likely to ever be involved.

Here are the Zodiac signs and the body parts they govern:

Sign	Health issue
Aries	head, brain
Taurus	neck, throat, ears, nose, teeth
Gemini	lungs
Cancer	skin
Leo	heart, blood
Virgo	food intake intestines
Libra	food processing intestines
Scorpio	genitals
Sagittarius	eyes
Capricorn	bones, spine
Aquarius	arms, legs
Pisces	nerves

Be aware that your horoscope cares little about what substances you're actually allergic to. It shows instead how your body reacts, and how it affects your life.

Look at the 12th House in your horoscope. If its Zodiac sign governs body parts prone to show some allergy symptoms, you may be sensitive to that specific allergy. That's particularly plausible if you have planets in the House – especially the sun, Mercury or Jupiter, which are the most likely to create allergy there.

Those planets don't need to be in the 12th House to cause allergy, but if they are elsewhere, they must be badly aspected or obstructed in some other way. Also the 6th House might cause allergy in the body part governed by its Zodiac sign, but probably not without the sun, Mercury or Jupiter in it – whether badly aspected or not.

Whatever House the planet causing the allergy is in, it's the Zodiac sign it occupies that decides the type of allergy – what body part it will harass.

Transits are unlikely to create allergy, but they may trig-

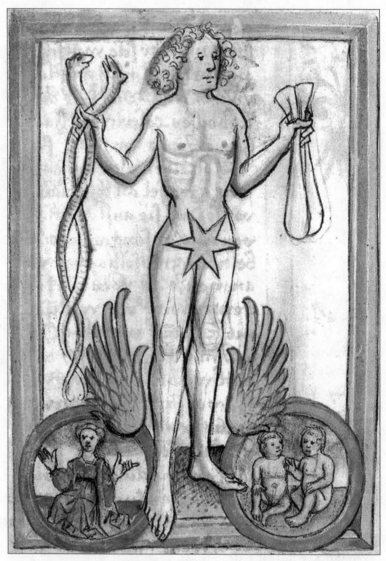

Mercury and the signs where the planet rules and exalts. Book illumi-
nation from 1429.

Your Health in Your Horoscope

ger a dormant one, or make a mild allergy worse. Since that's usually a lasting thing, it has to be one of the slower planets – most likely Jupiter or Saturn – and in a transit opposition, square, or conjunction. If it's a square, the allergy will not last as long and be as severe as if it's one of the other two aspects.

When you have located the allergy in your horoscope you can treat it, maybe even cure it, by stimulating the native planet involved, so that obstructions to it are eased. Check other aspects to it – or to a planet conflicting it – and ponder how to make their forces work more smoothly.

For example, if you have Mercury in the 12th House and Cancer, and suffer allergic rash of some kind, take a look at any aspects Mercury might have to other planets in your horoscope. They are the reasons Mercury is held back, which is what causes the allergy. Try to allow Mercury to act anyway – in this case by expressing your feelings verbally. Let people know, and adjust your everyday life accordingly. Speak out whenever you feel the need. Communicate with others, even if it's time-consuming and you seem not to reach them.

When Mercury is stimulated, it will cease just yielding to the aspected planets and not react with allergy. Even if Mercury has no aspect to other planets, you should stimulate it in order to treat your allergy – but in that case it is more difficult for you to find ways to express your Mercury properly.

When the planet causing your allergy is elsewhere than in the 12th House you should not really stimulate it, but almost the opposite. Allergy can be a result of over-stimulation, especially in the case of Jupiter and Mercury. So, if this can be suspected (by the planet being involved in a lot of other activity), try to tone it down, and transfer some attention to any other planets it may be aspected to.

Allergy is treated by balancing, which sometimes means more and sometimes less.

Blood pressure

The blood, as well as the heart, is governed by Leo. If Leo is in the 12th House, there is a risk that you have a heart weaker than you want it to be. As for your blood pressure, it's most likely to be low with Leo in that House – if you don't have the sun, Mars or Jupiter there. In that case it may be high.

Regarding the condition of the heart and blood, Leo is what to watch the closest. If Leo is in one of the Houses that are expansive and active by nature, the blood pressure is more likely to be high than low. They are: 1st, 3rd, 5th, 7th, 9th, and 11th. These Houses correspond to the air and fire Zodiac signs. The other Houses correspond to earth and water.

As for the planets, some are more likely to cause high blood pressure than the others. They are the sun, Mars, and Jupiter. But any active planets in Leo easily result in high blood pressure and some additional strain on the heart, especially if they have aspects to other planets stimulating or obstructing them.

Transiting planets don't really cause changes to the blood pressure directly. But if they point to planets in Leo, they can cause intensified activity, which is likely to raise the blood pressure. Mars can do that just by passing through Leo, or the signs in square to it: Taurus and Scorpio. To a lesser extent, that's true for the sun as well.

Such blood pressure rises are troublesome if your Leo is additionally complicated – like when it's in the 12th House, or contains planets in obstructing aspects with other planets in the horoscope.

If your Leo is void of planets, and placed in a House

with an even number, you may have low blood pressure. That's likely also if you have the moon in Leo, or to a lesser extent Neptune.

Obesity

Obesity is far from always a disease in any way, but it can be. Some people gain weight even when their eating habits are reasonable, and others are compulsive eaters. In those cases, it makes sense to regard obesity as a kind of disease or ailment.

If obesity is caused by some kind of nutritional problem or one of digestion and metabolism, the astrological cause is likely to be found in Virgo or Libra. The former governs the early food processing, like the stomach, and the latter governs the later process of the intestines.

If either of the signs is in the 12th House, some food processing disorder is likely. If also the expansive planet Jupiter is there, or Venus or the sun, there is a risk of obesity. In many cases the problem is simply that you don't allow your eating and metabolism the peace and quiet necessary. Too often, there is not enough time, because of other commitments in life.

If such planets in the 12th House have obstructing aspects to other planets in the horoscope, the problem is more complicated. You need to consider exactly what in life interferes with your eating and food processing, in order to balance the situation. For example, you should absolutely try to eat at times when the activities of those aspecting planets are at rest.

Obesity as a problem for your appearance is shown mainly by the Ascendant, maybe also by a square from Medium Coeli to it. If the Ascendant is in an earth sign (Taurus, Virgo, or Capricorn) there is some risk of getting an

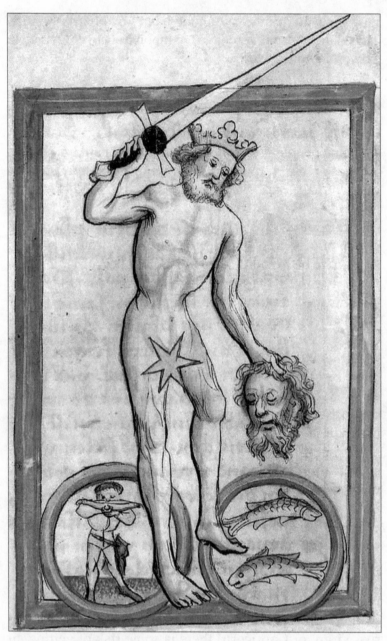

Jupiter with the ruling and exalting signs. Book illumination from 1429.

Your Health in Your Horoscope

obese appearance, especially if Jupiter, the sun or Venus is conjunct to it – in some cases also if there is a sextile or a square.

Overall, the earth signs of the Zodiac are the ones to watch the closest, when it comes to obesity and other health conditions increasing the body weight.

Ulcer

Gastric ulcer relates to the stomach, which is governed by Virgo. If this sign is in your 12th House, you are likely to be sensitive to ulcer, so you should take extra care about your diet and your eating habits. This is particularly true if you have Mars or Saturn in the same House, or if other planets in the House have obstructive aspects to planets elsewhere in the horoscope.

But whatever House Virgo occupies, there is a risk for gastric ulcer if the environment of that House is troubled. For example, if you have Virgo in the 4th House you are likely to feel stomach aches in times of family trouble, and if it's in the 6th House you get it when you have a hard time at work.

Here are the environments of the Houses that may lead to stomach trouble with Virgo in them, when conflicted or strained:

House	Keyword
1st House	*Identity*. How others see you.
2nd House	*Resources*. Your personal ability and economy.
3rd House	*Communication*. Your friends and acquaintances, also education.
4th House	*Home*. Your home and family.
5th House	*Pastime*. Your personal preferences, pleasures and interests.

6th House	*Work*. Your profession and daily work.
7th House	*Partners*. Your partners in love and other relations.
8th House	*Unknown*. What you cannot control – fate as well as bloodline.
9th House	*Travel*. Changes of your perspective.
10th House	*Career*. Your social status.
11th House	*Ideals*. Your ideals, and your interaction in the community.
12th House	*Shortcomings*. Your sacrifices, what you are unable to express.

Normally, you don't need astrology to see this relation between the House, Virgo, and your stomach ache. If you manage to solve the troublesome issue of the House, your stomach ache is also likely to pass – unless Virgo is additionally burdened by Mars, Saturn, or Pluto, or obstructive aspects to other planets in the sign.

But even in those cases, which are more severe, your stomach trouble is somewhat eased by solving troublesome issues of the House.

Diabetes

Diabetes is a metabolism malfunction that can be very troublesome, and easily fatal if neglected. The fact that it is caused by faulty metabolism suggests the Zodiac sign Libra, which governs the food processing functions of the body, but astrology is more about effect than cause. The horoscope shows how ailments affect your life, not necessarily what biochemistry lies behind them.

In the case of diabetes, you will need to keep a strict balance in your diet – or between your intake of sugar and injected insulin. This emphasis on balance again suggests

Libra, the very sign of balance, and of keeping a middle course.

For the above two reasons combined, diabetes must be regarded as a Libra ailment.

Of course, with Libra in your 12th House there is a higher risk of developing diabetes – at childhood or later on. The same is true for the 8th House, since this ailment can be immediately fatal if not treated constantly. It might even be true for the 6th House, if your work somehow strains your metabolism or makes you neglect a sound diet.

But it's not enough to have Libra in one of those Houses. Some planet has to be involved, in order for this serious ailment to erupt. Because of the expansive biochemical nature of diabetes in your body, and how it messes up your balances, Jupiter is likely to be involved. It's also powerful enough. But Jupiter is normally a benevolent planet, so it has to be heavily obstructed or disturbed by other planets.

The seriousness and persistence of the ailment points to Saturn being involved. Not that a native Saturn in Libra would cause diabetes. It would strike in a more evident and less subtle way. But a transit Saturn in Libra could do it, also Saturn in an obstructive aspect with a planet in Libra, especially if that sign is in the 12th, 8th, or 6th House. The risk is higher if that planet is Jupiter or the sun.

The hidden character of diabetes, such as the fact that it's deadly although there's no visible sign of it, also suggests Scorpio. Scorpio has a lot to do with the body's biochemistry, its enzymes and other inner workings. So, the above planetary ingredients might lead to diabetes also in Scorpio. But one of those planets would need to be of a lighter character than Saturn or Pluto. Otherwise the ailment would be more visible and concrete. Jupiter could be such a planet. Maybe the sun, and maybe even Mercury.

Mercury is not unlikely to lie behind the emergence of diabetes, because of the subtle way of its working. But the planet is rarely that malicious, so it needs to be obstructed by a more powerful one – most likely Saturn or Pluto.

There is not yet a cure for diabetes, so once it has emerged it is chronic. This points to Saturn and Pluto, certainly. Those grim planets also explain why it is fatal if neglected even the slightest.

I see no easy way to treat it astrologically. If it's based in Libra it is obvious that one must respect the balance. If the trigger is a planet outside Libra forming an obstructive aspect with a planet in that sign, then the symptoms and complications of diabetes can be softened by paying attention to that planet and its demands – also to the planet in Libra, and how it can be expressed in a positive way.

But mainly, the balance needs to be kept.

If the ailment is based in Scorpio, any treatment of it is even more difficult. Paying attention to outside planets aspecting a planet in Scorpio might be easy, but to stimulate a planet in the sign is often tricky, because it is hard to understand how to express it. Scorpio is the sign of the suppressed and hidden. It will not reveal itself at just any request.

Such a situation needs to be meditated. Generally speaking, stimulating a Scorpio situation involves accepting urges from deep within.

Arthritis

Arthritis strikes the joints, which are governed by Aquarius. Gemini might also be involved, regarding the agility of the hands and fingers. If one of those signs is in the 12th House, there may be a risk of getting arthritis, mainly in the hands if it's Gemini, whereas Aquarius can strike the hands as well as the rest of the body.

Your Health in Your Horoscope

The same is true for the 6th House, especially after many years of hard work.

Aquarius and Gemini may lead to arthritis even in other Houses, if either of the signs contains Mars or Saturn. These two are the most likely planets to cause this ailment, especially if they are obstructed by aspects to other planets in strong positions.

Arthritis can cause quite some pain, which connects it to Mars and Saturn. The former usually leads to short periods of intense pain, while the latter mostly means long periods of ache. Both can be instrumental in the deformities of some serious cases of arthritis.

The ailment is most common among old people. This points to Pluto, the last of the planets, particularly connected to the end of our years. So, Pluto can also cause the development of arthritis, especially among seniors, either by occupying Aquarius or Gemini in the birth chart, or by obstructive aspects to planets in those signs – whether that is in the birth chart or as a transit later on in life.

All three planets are severe, so ailments introduced by them are difficult to heal, even more so if they have a troublesome position in the birth chart. But the pain and suffering can be eased by compensating for the obstruction the planets may cause, or by being sensitive to what they need to express if they are in Aquarius or Gemini.

AIDS

In the beginning of November 1983, Pluto entered Scorpio, the sign ruled by that planet. Since Pluto wasn't discovered until 1930, this was the first time we could observe its entry into that sign – the one where the planet is the strongest.

Scorpio governs the genitals and sexuality, so it could be no surprise that the disease AIDS surfaced at about that

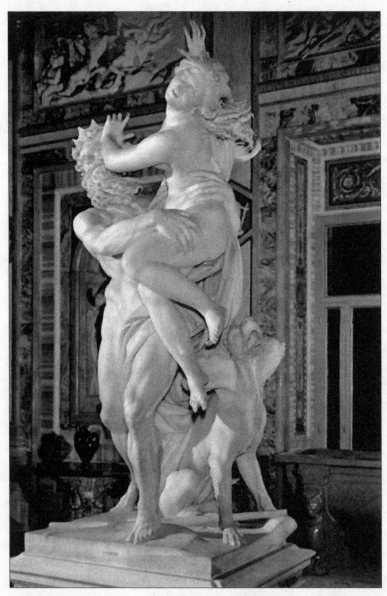

Pluto's rape of Prosperine. Statue by Gian Lorenzo Bernini, 1622. Pluto was the god of the netherworld in Roman mythology, inherited from Greek mythology where he was called Hades.

Your Health in Your Horoscope

time. Therefore we know that AIDS is very much linked to Pluto in Scorpio. It makes no difference that the disease is actually older than that, since it didn't erupt and create a crisis until the 1980's.

Pluto's relevance to AIDS is also evident in the fact that it's a lethal disease, and Pluto is indeed of that magnitude. The planet is closely connected to death, since it's the horoscope's symbol of the passage into that realm.

Pluto left Scorpio in 1995, after 12 years. That's unusually quick for Pluto, which takes 248 years to go through the whole Zodiac. Because of its elliptic orbit, it is the quickest in its ruling sign Scorpio.

So, the crisis of AIDS in society should have ceased after 1995, which doesn't mean that it ceased to exist as a disease. But cures had been introduced, and AIDS was no longer threatening to cause genocide.

On the other hand it should be noted that all the people born with Pluto in Scorpio are at heightened risk to get the disease. That was clear when it struck many children, even newborn ones, already early after its appearance.

Individual sensitivity to AIDS can be seen in the position of Pluto in your personal horoscope. If it's afflicted by bad aspects to other planets, or if it's in the 12th or the 8th House, there's an additional risk that you might get it – especially if you're born with the planet in Scorpio.

On the other hand, if your Pluto is in another House, and not obstructed by aspects to other powerful planets, you are unlikely to catch the disease.

However: since effective medication against the disease has been introduced, its effect on people's lives has changed. Therefore, it's no longer necessarily so that AIDS will show through Pluto in your horoscope. If you get HIV, your horoscope chart will show it where it affects your life the most. Probably in the 7th House, showing your partnership, which is quite certain to be gravely affected by the disease.

Transits must also be observed. Transit Pluto, of course, can introduce the risk of HIV contamination, if coming in a malicious aspect to your sun, or another important point in your native chart. Saturn might do the same, but that's highly unlikely.

You should also pay attention to Scorpio, the sign linked to AIDS. If you have it in your 12th House, you may be particularly vulnerable to HIV and to other sexually transmitted diseases. That's also true for Scorpio in the 8th House. If Scorpio is in the 5th or 7th House there is also an increased risk, because you tend to take chances in your sex life.

This is a Pluto thing, and a Scorpio setting, so those are the major ingredients to observe.

Star health horoscopes

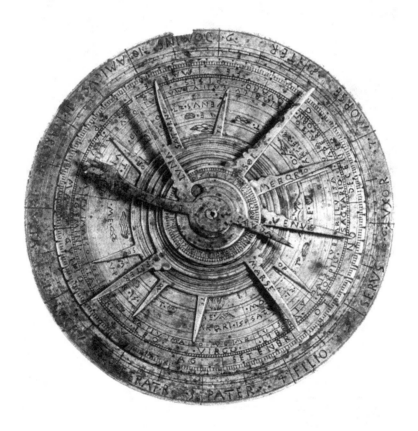

Astrolabe, an instrument for calculating the positions of the celestial bodies, made out of brass, from the late 15th century.

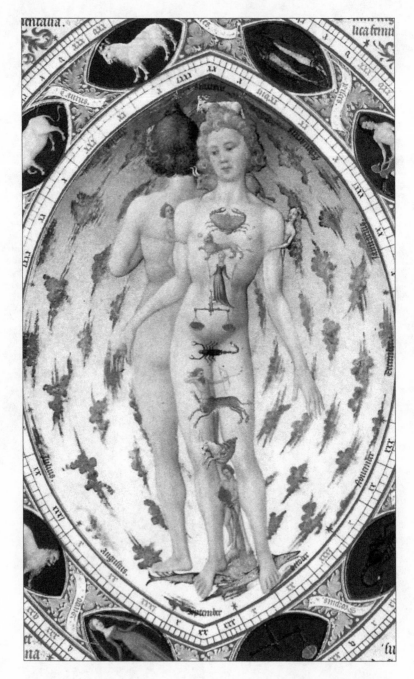

Your Health in Your Horoscope

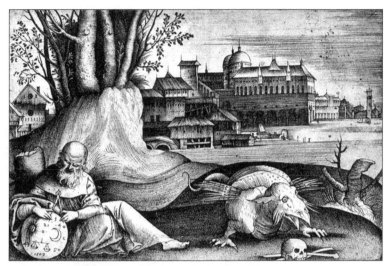

Astrologer. Etching by Giulio Campagnola, 1509.

Star health horoscopes

Below, I've had a glance at the horoscopes of a few famous people, to see what their charts say about their health. I don't go that very deep into those charts, nor have I picked them for any particular reason. They just serve as examples of how medical astrology can be applied to personal horoscopes.

As far as I know, the birth data of the below celebrities are somewhat ascertained. Still, it's always wise to be in some doubt about such things. Therefore, don't regard either the charts or my interpretations below as guaranteed. Whether the birth data are to be trusted or not, these horoscopes serve as examples of how one's health can be explored through one's horoscope.

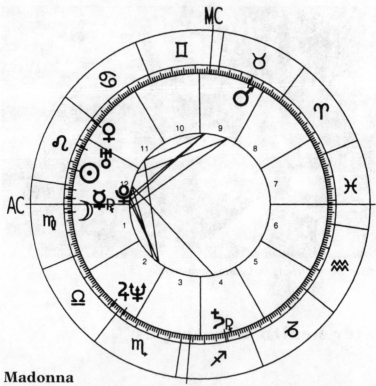

Madonna

As far as we know from the media, Madonna's health seems
to be fine. According to her horoscope, this can't be completely true. She has four planets in the 12th House, which is
the House of weaknesses and sacrifice. Even her sun, the
most important indicator of a person's health, is in that
House.

It's in the Zodiac sign Leo, which governs the heart and
the blood. Since Madonna's sun is rather late in Leo, on the
23rd of its 30 degrees, it has to do more with the blood than
with the heart. That's the mutable decan of the sign, indicating the blood floating through the body. The heart is more
connected to the cardinal decan of the sign, its first ten
degrees, since the heart is the power that actually pumps the
blood.

With that position of the sun, Madonna is very likely to have some kind of problem with her blood. For example, high blood pressure is quite likely. Whatever the specific condition, its effect is one of fatigue. It is tiresome to her, so she has to find methods to compensate for it in order to keep her stamina up.

The sun's aspects are a sextile to Jupiter in the 2nd House, and a trine to Saturn in the 4th. That means Madonna's blood problems are caused by her wealth and her difficulties in handling family matters as she should. That sounds like pressure, so it's quite likely that she has blood pressure problems.

By the end of the 12th House, she has Pluto and Mercury, not close enough to melt into one. Both of them are in Virgo, the sign that commences at the end of the House. That indicates some serious complications with her food intake, and a necessity for Madonna to be very picky about what she eats. Otherwise her stomach is at risk.

Pluto is a very grave power in the horoscope, especially in this House, so she is wise to respect its warning signals. Mercury indicates that she is sensitive to these signals and adapts to them, although reluctantly. Sometimes she can get a bit over-concerned. Well, better safe than sorry.

Apart from the above, there are no real threats to Madonna's health in the horoscope. Saturn in Sagittarius is retrograde, which makes it frustrated but also weakened. It may cause some complications to her vision, especially when she is under strain, and some ache in connection to that. Maybe she is too stubborn to wear glasses although she should.

Mars in the middle of Taurus in the 9th House is sort of a paradox. The 9th House stands for change, and Taurus for continuity. So, through her life changes Madonna insists on continuity. Mars brings some intensity to this conflict, but it also gives her the strength to solve it, sometimes in quite a drastic way.

Still, in times of change Madonna may react with sudden Taurus symptoms: trouble with the nose, throat, ears, and teeth. Maybe she gnaws her teeth when having to shift habits she would prefer to keep, for example. Mars in Taurus would trigger something like that, when obstructed.

I have to finish by expressing some doubt about Madonna's birth time. Leo is the sign of personal success and pride. The fist part of it is at the end of the 11th House, which deals with fame, and on the very first grade of Leo is Venus, giving pleasure and progress. But can Madonna really have so much of Leo in the 12th House, the one of sacrifice and the unfulfilled?

Her given birth time, 7:05 AM, might be a bit off. I would be more convinced by a slightly later birth time, putting most of Leo in her 11th House, and most of her 1st House in Libra rather than Virgo. Madonna's ascendant might still be Virgo, the Virgin, which was the archetype she played with when she introduced herself to the world.

If she was indeed born a little later than 7:05, most of the above would still be true. Actually, her health issues would not change much, even if she was born as much as an hour later.

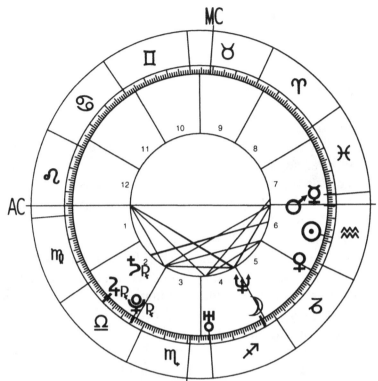

Justin Timberlake

We move on to another pop star, who has actually cooper-
ated recently with Madonna. Justin Timberlake has a very
interesting horoscope, because almost all of its ingredients
are below the horizon – in the 1st to 6th Houses. That semi-
circle of the chart is the private side, whereas Houses 7 to 12
are the public ones.

Why would a boy who got world famous already as a
child have so little happening in the public half of his chart?
We need to remain in some doubt about Justin Timberlake's
birth time, although it is reported to be confirmed by a birth
certificate or some similar evidence. Also, 6:30 PM is a bit
too even to be real. 6:29 or 6:31 would have been easier to
believe.

Anyway, we work on what we have.

Justin actually has his 12th House in Leo, like Madonna. Even more so, since just 5 degrees of the sign are outside the House. But in his case, there are no planets in that House, so he might have some problems with his heart or the blood, but they are not likely to be severe.

Both his Mars and his sun are in Aquarius and the 6th House – although Mars is less than half a degree from the 7th House, so it's really to be regarded as on it cusp. Aquarius governs the arms and legs, as well as their movements. Justin Timberlake has shown by his dancing that he can work with those.

His sun even implies that he's more of a dancer than a singer, but it also shows that he can have trouble with his limbs when he gets tired, or when his sun is obstructed in some way. It's not very likely to happen, though, since its only aspect is the trine to his conjunction of Jupiter and Saturn in Libra and the 2nd House.

That trine also preserves Justin Timberlake from problems with the very strong conjunction of those two planets. Otherwise, they could easily lead to severe complications in his food processing organs. Since this conjunction is shared by most people born the same year, many others will surely suffer such health issues during periods of their lives. Not Justin.

He has another conjunction, which could also cause health issues: that of Neptune and the moon in Sagittarius, at the end of his 4th House. Obstructed or held back, it would surely lead to a loss of his sense of reality. But Justin has two sextiles and one trine to other planets in his chart, so he should do fine. He has many means to express this conjunct power, which is most certainly the source to his creativity – flowing inspiration and artistic vision.

Justin Timberlake's ascendant is in an almost exact

opposition to the aforementioned Mars. It shows that he often has to put his personality aside for the sake of his relation to a partner. That could lead to some grumpy behavior, but hardly any kind of disease.

So, Justin Timberlake is quite a healthy person, who can expect to escape serious illnesses or other health problems of any dignity. The most serious threat to his health was when transit Pluto formed a Square aspect to his native sun, which was in the year 2000. Evidently, he managed that astral crisis, so he can relax.

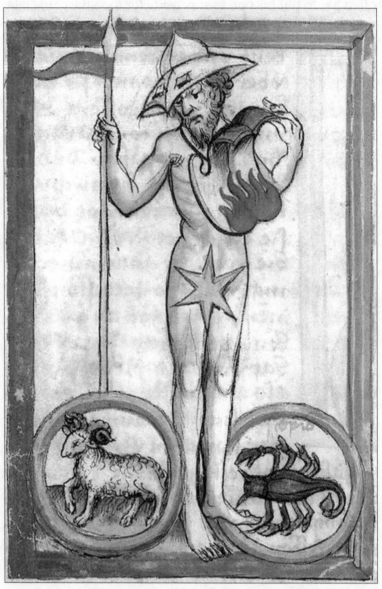

Mars and the signs where the planet rules and exalts. Book illumination from 1429.

Your Health in Your Horoscope

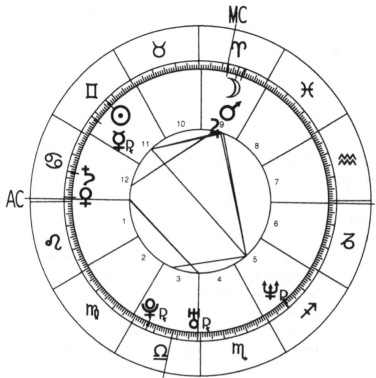

Angelina Jolie

I trust Angelina Jolie's birth time more than the ones above. It's given as 9:09 AM, which is odd enough to be to the point, and her chart makes a lot of sense.

Her 1st House is indeed Leo, what else could it be? Her ascendant is Cancer, but at its very end, only slightly more than one degree from Leo, so it just adds an emotional flare to Angelina Jolie's Leo appearance. As many as 29 of the sign's 30 degrees are in the 1st House.

Venus is in conjunction with Angelina Jolie's ascendant, which accounts for her charisma. She also has the sun in the 11th House, indicating fame, and a bunch of planets in the 9th House and Leo, showing her ability to "conquer the world," and some other ingredients explaining her success.

But here, we are interested in what Angelina Jolie's horoscope says about her health. Her 12th House is in Cancer, the sign that governs the skin, so she may have some problem in that area. It can be severe at times, because Saturn is in that House, which is a particularly frustrating position for that planet. A frustrated Saturn can cause serious and lasting problems.

Saturn has a square aspect to the powerful conjunction of MC and Jupiter in the 9th House and Aries – a conjunction that generally makes her able to intentionally accomplish great changes in her life, all of them for the better. But the square to Saturn introduces complications, so Angelina Jolie might have a skin condition that can get triggered by drastic changes she makes in her life, and this health issue sometimes risks standing in the way of such changes.

But the conjunction of MC and Jupiter is too powerful to yield to Saturn in the 12th House. So, things work out every time, although Angelina Jolie might need to do some adaptions to the needs Saturn creates. Because MC, her self-awareness, is also in square to Saturn, she is probably reluctant to accept that weakness. This resistance of hers can cause increasing problems, especially at length.

Angelina's sun is in Gemini and the 11th House, indicating her fame as an entertainer. It has a sextile aspect to Mars and the moon in the 9th House, showing that the changes in her life increase her fame. But the sun is also in opposition to Neptune in her 5th House, which means that her fame stands in the way of her dreams of freedom and independence, the impulse to leave everything else, just to indulge in her own fantasies.

This opposition can cause some Gemini type health issues – expressed in her breathing or speech. But the sextile to the 9th House makes this rather unlikely. Mars and the moon in that House also have a trine to Neptune, which releases the tension of the opposition, and explains it: In order to accomplish the big changes in her life, Angelina Jolie needs both her fame and her fantasies.

The center of her horoscope is the 9th House, with its two powerful conjunctions. Change of an often adventurous nature is what drives her – not fame. If she tries to hold that urge back, she will get severe headaches and a frustration that can escalate quite quickly.

Angelina Jolie's Pluto is in Libra, which she shares with her whole generation, but also in the 3rd House, and that's personal to her. It can cause sudden changes of what friends she has, often for moral reasons, but it is not likely to cause her some specific health problems.

Actually, apart from the skin problem, Angelina Jolie is quite healthy.

That skin problem follows the cycles of Saturn, so it is intensified every 14 to 15 years, when transit Saturn moves into opposition or conjunction with it. Her skin condition may enter a new phase, maybe much more serious, when transit Pluto moves into opposition with it, which is in the year 2017.

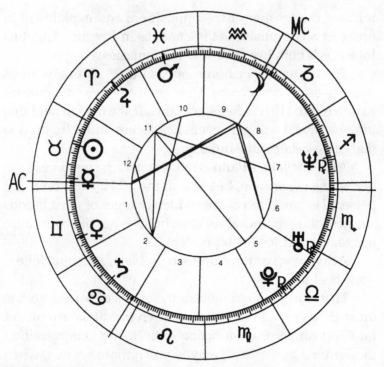

David Beckham

The birth time of the world-famous soccer player David Beckham seems quite trustworthy. It's realistically uneven, 6:17 AM, and the chart contains some plausible ingredients – such as Jupiter in Aries and the 11th House, indicating fame through success in challenging ways, like sports. Fame is something he wins.

As for David Beckham's health, his 12th House is in Taurus, which makes for weaknesses in his throat, ears, and nose. He is likely to easily catch a cold. His sun is in that House, so his Taurus weaknesses are something he just has to live with. The sun has no troublesome aspect, though. Therefore it is improbable that he gets very serious problems – but conditions in his throat, ears, or nose will repeatedly fatigue him.

In the summer of 1988, when he was just 13, David Beckham had some health crisis related to the Taurus organs. It was when transit Pluto formed an opposition aspect to his sun. Pluto did so in Scorpio and Beckham's 6th House, which suggests that the problems were related to serious threats in his work. Surely, his work was already at that time soccer more than school or anything else. He will not experience any such serious threat to his health again.

Apart from the above, I don't see much of health problems in David Beckham's horoscope. He has a nice spread of planets, so there's no particular cluster that he needs to be wary of.

Saturn in Cancer and his 2nd House might occasionally cause some skin irritations, especially when David Beckham's fame makes him neglect duties he has to himself personally. But that is probably never serious or lasting.

Mars is in Pisces, which is the sign where Mars is the least comfortable. That might lead to occasional nervousness, and instants of a short temper that seems to be completely uncalled for. Again, probably never serious.

That's about it. Every athlete should be this healthy, but few are.

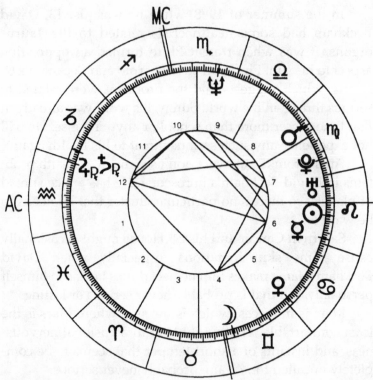

Barack Obama

The birth time of Barack Obama is ascertained by his birth certificate being published during his presidential campaign, for some political reason. He was born on August 4, 1961, at 7:24 PM in Honolulu. That's precise enough to be very trustworthy.

Similar to some of the other horoscopes mentioned above, Obama's 12th House is heavily burdened. The grim planet Saturn is there, and so is Jupiter. Both of them tend to be kind of frustrated in that House, so they are likely to create health issues. But both are in retrograde, which softens their force, and therefore also their potential danger.

Retrograde is when a planet seems to be moving backward in the sky, as seen from Earth. That's because Earth moves as well, so in parts of its orbit around the sun, another planet observed from here can give that impression. It happens to all the planets, but never to the sun or the moon.

Both Saturn and Jupiter are obstructed just by being in retrograde, but so is their malicious power. Still, in the 12th House, bad consequences to the health should be expected.

They occupy one Zodiac sign each. Saturn, the most complicated of the two, is in the third decan of Capricorn, indicating some problems with the bones. Obama probably has a hazardous or complicated weakness in his bones, already from birth. It is more likely to cause trouble with the smaller bones of his body, and the surface of them, than with the biggest and strongest bones of his body. The spine is probably not affected.

Saturn has a benevolent trine to Mars in his 8th House and Virgo, which eases his trouble. It suggests that he was born with a strength to forebear the trouble his bone weakness might cause. But it's a delicate balance, so he should avoid putting strain on his bone structure. For example, it's good that he is far from overweight. Mars in Virgo indicates a metabolism that makes him unlikely to gain weight, even if he eats a lot.

Jupiter is almost at the cusp of Aquarius, less than one degree into the sign. That deals with the limbs, the arms and legs, which is also something connected to the bone structure. Obama might occasionally lose control of his limbs, as if they are too much to handle. He needs to keep his body movements rather restricted for this not to show.

Jupiter has an opposition to Venus in his 6th House and Leo, showing that this weakness is particularly troublesome for him in doing his job, where he needs to present himself as particularly able. But there is also a trine to the moon in his 4th House and Gemini. It means that within his family,

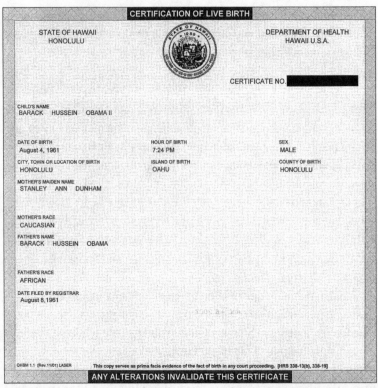

CERTIFICATION OF LIVE BIRTH

STATE OF HAWAII
HONOLULU

DEPARTMENT OF HEALTH
HAWAII U.S.A.

CERTIFICATE NO.

CHILD'S NAME
BARACK   HUSSEIN   OBAMA II

DATE OF BIRTH
August 4, 1961

HOUR OF BIRTH
7:24 PM

SEX
MALE

CITY, TOWN OR LOCATION OF BIRTH
HONOLULU

ISLAND OF BIRTH
OAHU

COUNTY OF BIRTH
HONOLULU

MOTHER'S MAIDEN NAME
STANLEY   ANN   DUNHAM

MOTHER'S RACE
CAUCASIAN

FATHER'S NAME
BARACK   HUSSEIN   OBAMA

FATHER'S RACE
AFRICAN

DATE FILED BY REGISTRAR
August 8,1961

QHBM 1.1 (Rev.11/01) LASER   This copy serves as prima facie evidence of the fact of birth in any court proceeding. [HRS 338-13(b), 338-19]

ANY ALTERATIONS INVALIDATE THIS CERTIFICATE

Barack Obama's birth certificate.

Obama finds the support and comfort that protects him from mishaps because of his vulnerability. His wife is good at protecting him, as was his mother during his upbringing.

Obama's 6th House is divided between Cancer and Leo, but the two planets in the latter make that sign the most important one. As long as his work goes fine, and he is able to do it the way he wants to, there should be no health problem – but when that is not the case, he might get a galloping heartbeat as well as heightened blood pressure.

His Mars in Virgo mentioned above is in the 8th House, which may indicate some serious health issues. That would be the stomach and digestion. Normally, it works fine, but at length – especially when he gets older – serious problems can appear. An ulcer is not unlikely, especially when he feels that fate doesn't work in his favor.

His horoscope shows clearly that Barack Obama doesn't have an easy life. He must expect health problems, also some serious ones. Exactly how serious is difficult to say, but occasionally enough to demand his full attention, and sometimes even very hazardous to his well-being. But it's also clear that he will not let such things stop him.

At the time of his shouldering the presidency, transit Saturn was in conjunction with his Mars, which must have taken its toll on his stomach condition. And that's likely to be a lasting ailment, at least until August 2009, since that's when Saturn makes its final passing over Mars this time. It will not return there until almost 30 years later.

Far into the future, in the year 2020, transit Saturn reaches Saturn in his birth chart. That's a very serious time for him, where his health is greatly at risk, and there's not much he can do about it. And Pluto is in the vicinity, too, meeting with his native Saturn the following year. It's very much of a burden to carry, enough to make a man stumble and fall. But that's way ahead.

CPSIA information can be obtained
at www.ICGtesting.com
Printed in the USA
BVHW030900080121
597355BV00006B/53